PRAISES FOR

CIA Street Smarts for Women

"Part intelligence operative handbook—part *Mars & Venus*, B. D. Foley's *CIA Street Smarts* sparkles with hilarious stories, old-fashioned fatherly advice, and brilliant secret agent ideas for the woman who is trying to size up suitors and keep herself safe. The intrigue of Mr. Foley's real-life spy experiences and the warmth of his wisdom will help turn naïve schoolgirls into street-smart women."

—Karen Nickl, PhD, psychologist

"I served with Foley in the CIA, and he knows of what he speaks when it comes to traditional espionage tradecraft and staying alive in dangerous parts of the world. This book brings his experience to bear on a very topical subject: the safety and security of women in today's increasingly violent world. Utilizing the operational security, awareness techniques, and vetting mechanisms that many of us in the intelligence community have used for years to keep safe, even in our post-Agency careers, Foley brings down-to-earth and practical security tradecraft tips for not just women, but anyone who wants to be safer in this world and minimize the chances they will run afoul of bad people. There are many books out there written by former CIA officers, and each has its own merits and kudos to anyone who served in the Agency and helped to keep America safe. And now, kudos to Foley, for bringing his experience to bear to help keep women safe and secure. This is a very different optic when it comes to how to use traditional espionage tradecraft to keep civilians, in this case, women, safe. Definitely worth reading."

—Mike Howard, chief security officer, Microsoft Corporation

Mary,
Wish you the best!
BD Foley

Plain Sight Publishing

An imprint of Cedar Fort, Inc. • Springville, UT

CIA
Street Smarts
for women

spy skills to tell the
prince
from the
predator

B. D. Foley
retired CIA operations officer

All statements of fact, opinion, or analysis expressed are those of the author and do not reflect the official positions or views of Cedar Fort, Inc., the CIA, or any other US Government agency. Nothing in the contents should be construed as asserting or implying US Government authentication of information or Agency endorsement of the author's views. This material has been reviewed by the CIA to prevent the disclosure of classified information.

Permission for the use of sources, graphics, and photos is also solely the responsibility of the author.

ISBN: 978-1-4621-1768-0

Published by Plain Sight Publishing, an imprint of Cedar Fort, Inc.,
2373 W. 700 S., Springville, UT 84663
Distributed by Cedar Fort, Inc., www.cedarfort.com

LIBRARY OF CONGRESS CATALOGING-IN-PUBLICATION DATA
Foley, B. D., 1958- author.
CIA street smarts for women : spy skills to tell the prince from the predator / B.D. Foley.
pages cm
Includes bibliographical references.
ISBN 978-1-4621-1768-0 (perfect bound : alk. paper)
1. Women--Crimes against--Prevention. 2. Self-defense for women. 3. Women--Life skills guides.
I. Title.
HV6250.4.W65F65 2015
646.7'7082--dc23
            2015024995

Cover design by Lauren Error
Cover design © 2015 by Lyle Mortimer
Edited by Eileen Leavitt

Printed in the United States of America

10 9 8 7 6 5 4 3 2 1

Printed on acid-free paper

To my daughter, Shana

Contents

1
Romantic Espionage

Tammy was my first love, and I was possibly her first spy. I loved her to the depths of my ten-year-old heart, which, granted, was not all that deep. She was all I thought of in fifth grade. On second thought, I also thought a lot about shooting marbles, building forts, and catching snakes, so maybe what I was feeling wasn't exactly love, but I found her to be fascinating and definitely worth watching.

And boy, did I watch that girl! I studied her every move during class, lunch, and recess. I memorized her hair, her eyes, and the way she walked and talked. I suppose all that attention would be interpreted these days as stalking but without the harassment or sinister intentions. When I look back, I would call it spying.

I didn't realize it at the time, but I was a born spy: surveilling and assessing her, identifying her likes and dislikes. With no training at all, I was gathering information, or—in spy terms—*intelligence*. What are her interests? Does she prefer the swings, monkey bars, or slippery slide? Tetherball or kickball? Pixie sticks or Smarties?

More important than *what* she liked was *whom* she liked. Or better yet, whom did she love? Particularly, did she love me? Did she know that I loved her? Did she want to play with me at recess? Where? When?

So many questions, and I had to know the answers. So I put my sources to work. Top-secret messages soon crisscrossed the classroom in the form of hand signals, nods, and winks. Cryptic notes were expertly passed from source to agent, fingertip to fingertip, under desktops, handled as professionally as any CIA operation. Most of the communication went undetected despite being transmitted under the nose of our teacher, whom we considered a member of the hostile intelligence agency.

One of my sources soon reported that he had successfully arranged a meeting with Tammy. She had agreed to talk with me next to the monkey bars during the next recess. Despite my strict warnings to keep it secret, however, word of the meeting soon leaked through the class. *Loose lips sink ships.*

When the time finally arrived, I was waiting at the appointed meeting site, nervous with anticipation, but hopeful. I watched as Tammy approached very slowly, her arms folded behind her back, black leather shoes clicking on the pavement. She was beautiful in her light pastel pink summer dress, which fluttered in the breeze. Her head bowed slightly, and she looked up at me with a subtle Mona Lisa smile.

The moment had arrived. All that spy work—targeting, surveillance, secret communications, OPSEC (operational security)—was now culminating in a covert meeting with my Bond girl. It was elementary school espionage at its finest—all for love.

But suddenly, as I waited for our meeting to begin, I noticed that she began to giggle. Why she would giggle at such a serious moment was beyond me. I was as serious as a heart attack. Actually, I was about to have a heart attack. And just as I began to ask "What the . . . ?" she turned and sprinted away. Her team of counter-surveillant friends all whirled as one, like a flock of birds following the lead sparrow, running and squealing with delight and fright.

Things do not always go according to plan in espionage. Instead of standing there next to her, maybe offering her a Pixie Stick and inviting her to shoot marbles, I was now watching her run away. And in an instant, I found myself running after her, not knowing what else to do. Running must be the default in a ten-year-old's brain. If all else fails, run.

I quickly gained on her, but as I closed the distance, she stopped suddenly and crouched down, maybe to buckle her shoe; why, I will never know. What I do know is I stepped on the hem of her dress just as she was rising again to her feet. The skirt portion tore away from the body of the dress, making a horrible ripping noise—a sound worse than fingernails on a chalkboard. The memory still makes me cringe.

Tammy reacted as if I had slapped her across the face. My team of sources, now filling the role of my counter-surveillants, all froze in shock and then instantly scattered in all directions, knowing it was time to escape and evade. Every man for himself!

Tammy's friends gathered around her as she cried, each one casting angry, indignant glares in my direction. I stood there alone and would have gladly disappeared in a puff of smoke or crawled into a crack in the pavement if I could.

Tammy's dress, along with all of my well-crafted spy plans, was in tatters. The op was up. A true intelligence disaster. And my cover was blown. News of the torn dress spread throughout the school like wildfire: "B. D. tore Tammy's dress. B. D. tore Tammy's dress." Everyone in our school, I am sure, now knew that I loved Tammy, and that she definitely did not love me.

Blown operations always make front-page news. No one ever hears of successes in espionage, only the disasters. None of my schoolmates remembered all the times that I had successfully met girls at the monkey bars, sharing Pixie Sticks, without incident. They would remember this one.

I was soon making the "perp walk" alone along the corridor to the principal's office—my head now bowed, hands behind my back, no need for handcuffs. The principal, the highest-ranking member of the hostile intelligence agency, seated behind his massive wooden desk, listed my charges: tearing Tammy's dress, conduct unbecoming an elementary school student. Punishment was swift: no recess for a week and a note to my parents. My mom, a member of the other hostile intelligence agency, gladly enforced additional, and far worse, consequences: mandatory shopping for a new dress and hand-delivery to Tammy's home.

I suspect that my mother did not know that delivering a dress to a girl, at ten years of age, was worse than torture. They could have pulled out my fingernails. Electrocution? Waterboarding? Come on. Those are nothing compared to being forced to shop for and deliver a dress to a girl's home.

The next day as I handed the dress to a grinning Tammy—yes, the Mona Lisa smile had been replaced by a full-bore smirk—on her front porch, I realized that not only was the operation over, so were we. We were done like a baked potato. Stick a fork in us. It was a very sad ending to a once promising relationship. I needed none of my sources to tell me the relationship was irreparable. No courtship could survive that kind of humiliation. Girls do not enjoy having their dresses torn. And boys especially do not like to shop.

Sure, I still noticed her from time to time from across the classroom, but I did not watch her anymore. I actually tried to not see her. Tammy was now just a former Bond girl, with all the others: Ursula Andress, Jane Seymour, Denise Richards, Halle Berry, and now Tammy. She was just another woman with a torn dress.

But although I had moved on and had terminated Tammy—in spy terms—my interest in spying was not over. This Bond had just moved on. And eighteen short years later, I found myself working for the ultimate spy agency, the Central Intelligence Agency (CIA), first as an analyst and then as an operations officer. I was now running sources for National Security rather than running after them on a playground for love. I was now a real, trained, bona fide spy.

I soon learned the skills associated with real spying: targeting and recruiting sources, eliciting intelligence, surveillance, and disguises. I learned the art of espionage, the craft, or *tradecraft*, as it is called in spy circles. Maybe "trade-crafty" would be a better description since spying is subtle, stealthy, and crafty.

I actually enjoyed espionage. But spying did not come particularly easy to me. I had to work at it, and I was determined. At the height of my career, I found myself trying to recruit practically everyone I met, everywhere I went: national day celebrations, volleyball matches, tennis tournaments, even at church. I worked at it so much during the day that I dreamed about it at night. I still do.

I tried not to step on any more dresses, so to speak, but I still made my share of missteps. I was once so determined in my pursuit of a diplomat from a former Soviet republic (let's call him Ivan) that I persuaded him to go golfing in the rain. He did not enjoy golf (neither did I), and especially not in the rain. After soaking for nine holes and listening to me repeat "the sun will come out any minute now!" Ivan was as irritated as he was wet. While I held the flag for him on the last green, he swung full force from a short distance away. I hardly saw the ball as it shot toward me and nailed me between the shoulder blades. I will never know if it was intentional. But as I sunk to my knees in pain, I noticed that his smile resembled Tammy's, from years earlier, when I handed her the new dress.

Another time, during a long, boring evening of "fishing" for sources at a European diplomatic function, I actually followed an undercover Chinese intelligence officer into a bathroom and introduced myself as we washed our hands at the sink. (Yes, I did that.) Again it was awkward, the results maybe more painful than Ivan's golf shot.

I console myself by knowing that nobody shoots 100 percent—not Lebron James nor James Bond. But I did succeed in many clandestine (secret) operations during my years in the CIA. And after a few decades of chasing people around the planet, I ended my career as an instructor, training a new generation of covert operations officers to take over the chasing.

Interestingly, through the years, I began to notice striking similarities between chasing Tammy and chasing spies. Both involve targeting tactics and stealthy pursuit of people, whether for national security or for the love of a classmate: surveillance, assessment, elicitation, vetting, and recruitment. I even encountered similar emotions tracking Tammy as zeroing in on a Russian officer of the KGB: excitement, anticipation, even perspiration.

And both espionage and romance have their seamy side. The artists of espionage and romance—predators—often resort to nefarious means to accomplish their goals: manipulation, plotting and planning, disguises, and lies. The target of a skilled covert intelligence agent is often unaware that she is being hunted. And the target of someone's affection, in the case of romance, can be just as oblivious. In both cases, the victims are often picked like a lemon, squeezed for information, or personal gratification, and discarded when of no further use. That may sound harsh and ruthless; it is.

Espionage and love seem to be inextricably bound together. Two sides of the same coin. Yin and yang. Espionage might be the second-oldest profession, but romance is the oldest preoccupation.

I understand some would argue that romance is not as serious a game as espionage and that the consequences of a romance gone wrong are not as severe. Granted, espionage is surely dangerous for all involved. I certainly risked my life on several occasions. Covert operations officers risk being captured or imprisoned. If officers choose the wrong target or are caught in clandestine acts, they could spend years in prison or even lose their lives.

But romance seems to be just as risky. Ask the families of heartbroken young women, abused girlfriends, or murdered wives if it is a serious game. When we really stop to consider the consequences of an intelligence failure in one's social life, it is obvious that the dating world can be just as perilous. A woman who chooses the wrong man, for instance, by dating a predator or encountering a stalker can face disastrous consequences. She can date wrong and even marry wrong and end up being abused or spending years in a loveless marriage. She might even lose her life.

Consider this—her choice of a man can alter her life for good or evil, for happiness or misery, for life or death. That is a long time. Romance and the choices she makes in that world is definitely no joke.

Given the level of potential damage to a young woman, I wonder why we have not been teaching skills—real spy skills—to help her navigate the iceberg-infested waters of romance.

Why aren't we training our young women in the art of romantic espionage at an early age? Shouldn't there at least be a class offered by the time she enrolls in college: Spy Skills for Ladies 101: a Beginning Course in Reading Men or How to Distinguish a Prince from a Toad, without All the Kissing. Maybe I will propose it to our local university.

I suspect that most young women take romance more seriously than men do. Men seem to be more cavalier about love, at least the ones that I have encountered over the years, including myself. Given a young woman's heightened concern, therefore, I am confident that she can become an artist in romantic espionage.

A woman with spy skills can learn to observe critically, listen carefully, be alert and careful in her surroundings, be discerning, and examine and test young men with the clarity and confidence of a spy.

A woman with spy skills can learn to recognize targeting techniques that young men might use against her and know when she is being manipulated. She can learn to identify a young man with bad intentions and "smell" him just as easily as I could smell an intelligence agent of the Russian KGB. And it wasn't due to the caviar on his breath.

Once a woman knows she is being targeted, she can take appropriate precautions and actions. She can remove herself from a potentially harmful encounter. She can avoid future contact with that person. She can avoid being in dangerous situations or associating with dangerous people in the future. Her increased knowledge and awareness can even help her avoid being targeted in the first place.

In short, a woman can avoid the Mr. Wrongs and then have the freedom to choose and recruit Mr. Right.

And that is the purpose of my book. There are enough movies, websites, books, and blogs on how to catch a man. I thought it only fair to teach a young lady how not to be caught, at least not by the wrong one.

This book is not really intended for a young man, unless he wants to learn what predators, stalkers, or plain, ordinary creeps do to young women and against women. Once a young man recognizes the manipulation and the hurt and heartache that predators cause women, then he might just decide that he does not want to be that guy. If that is the case, read on.

This book is also written for moms and dads of young women. I am writing on behalf of all those parents whose daughters do not listen to them often, if at all. If that is the case, then I hope these young ladies will listen to me because I am another daughter's dad.

2
Girls Are Precious

A Chapter for Dads

There are so many cycles in life. The cycle of water consists of evaporation, condensation, precipitation, and collection. The economic cycle follows this pattern: the economy improves, the stock market rises, the investor buys a boat, the economy crashes, and the stock market sinks . . . along with the boat. The cycle of a little girl begins when she is a helpless baby. She grows to toddlerhood, then breaks her dad's heart, then as a teenager breaks a young man's heart, and then as a wife breaks the suspension in the family car. (Yes, she did that.) The cycle of a little boy goes as follows: he's toothless and hairless, becomes a youth, becomes an adult, and then becomes an old man—again toothless and hairless. Not always, but often.

There is also the "How Men Perceive Women" cycle.

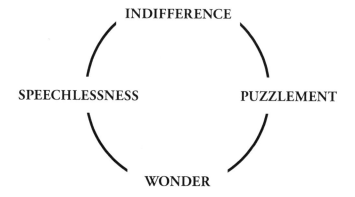

This cycle begins with *indifference*. A little boy cares little whether a playmate is male or female. All that matters is that the little girl will share her toys, is able to kick the ball back to him, and likes to play in a sand box. A little girl is someone with whom he plays, rides bikes, and swims, and who is just as good as any other child—no more, no less.

This indifference soon shifts to *puzzlement*. He notices that many little girls do not enjoy playing army in the sandbox or throwing dirt clods at each other during army games. Or squashing bugs. Or eating bugs. Girls often do not enjoy the same things boys do; they are strange that way.

He then feels *wonder* as he notices his sisters primping in front of the mirror. He learns that there must be something to a girl, given all the fuss.

And all that wonder causes him to watch. He starts spying on the little neighbor girl from a distance, from secret places in forts and tree houses. He sets up surveillance and an observation post (OP) in the bushes. He watches her riding down the street on her bike and notices how her hair blows in the wind (all that primping and brushing is paying off). He learns how to surveil the "girl with the golden hair," as my six-year-old son once called a classmate.

He watches, yes, but he also listens from a listening post (LP) in a tree next to her home, eavesdropping, or rather, leavesdropping. He pursues her, running around the neighborhood like James Bond, yes, but never quite getting the girl. He scrounges spy rings from cereal boxes and orders secret spy pens from comic books.

Then comes *speechlessness*. He would like to approach the little golden-haired girl and talk to her more than anything in the world, but he feels so much wonder that he cannot find the courage or the words. So he continues to watch, maybe no longer from up a tree, but from across the street, through his bedroom curtains, with the lights off to avoid detection, as she walks down the street. (Yes, I did that). He watches like a lion. A predator but without teeth.

The young man eventually notices that girls come in all shapes and sizes, like Legos, but now with more legs. All those female shapes lead not only to further deterioration of his vocabulary—breathless at beauty—but cold showers and sleepless nights.

He slowly learns to converse with his target, beginning with a one-word "hey," soon stringing a few more words together: "Hey, wassup?" Before long, he won't shut up, especially when the conversation shifts to new video games.

He is still spying now, but no more spy rings. In the blink of an eye, the little spy graduates to engagement ring, and puts a ring on her finger—as in the James Bond classic, *Goldfinger*. He is now that good at conversing, communicating, and persuading—at least good enough to convince her to marry him.

Unfortunately, at this point in the cycle, a man can devolve as quickly as he evolved, perhaps returning to his natural state—unable to communicate. And his vocabulary returns to the one-word "hey" or two-word "uh-huhs" or "uh-uhs," especially during an important football game (which is redundant, when you think about it). And the man-child might go from watching his foxy wife to watching Fox News.

Soon, a daughter is born to the couple, and he is now back to *wonder*. He wonders how that happened. He wonders how such a cute little girl could produce so many stinky diapers. But he also wonders at how beautiful his daughter is with her little nose and her almond eyes—a miniature version of his wife. He should stay at *wonder*.

But in another blink of an eye, he returns to *puzzlement*, because his beautiful little daughter has turned into a teenager. He is puzzled that his little girl can now drive a car. He is puzzled that she is so emotional. He has so many questions: Who is this girl? What did I say to upset her? Why does she cry so much? When did she grow up? Where did my little girl go?

His communication skills decompose further at this point. He now just watches his daughter rush in and out of the house to change clothes, eat, or sleep. He still tries to spy, to listen in on her phone conversations until she tells him to hang up the other phone. And then there is no other phone because she has her own cell phone. The eavesdropping drops and the conversation stops, except when she asks for money or the keys to the car.

The cycle continues throughout his life. A man often shifts through the four stages like gears of a car, unless he puts on the breaks.

Thankfully, a man has more choice than water or the economy in their cycles, and he does not have to continue full circle. He can keep communicating with his wife and daughter. He does not have to become puzzled—well, maybe a little—and especially not indifferent. He can even keep stringing multiple words together in a sentence.

A man can remain at wonder, as in amazement and awe. He can remember the wonder he felt at his daughter's birth, sixteen years earlier. He can remember her hugging his leg when he returned from work every

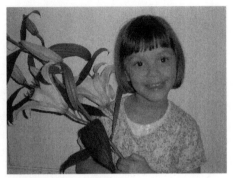

Our precious daughter.

day or sitting on his foot as he walked up the front steps and the paper neckties she made for Father's Day. He can wonder at her wonder when she sees a butterfly or a ladybug crawling on her finger. He can remember the hugs and the wonder.

A father can actually stay at the *wonder* stage.

"Tears, prayers, and flowers, you will do to my tomb, what I did at your cradle."[1] It is sad that we often do not appreciate someone until that person is gone—either on a trip, deceased, or even asleep. Maybe that's why a dad will go to his daughter's room at night, after she has gone to bed, sometimes to turn on her nightlight or pull her blankets around her chin to tuck her in. His daughter does not know that sometimes he sits beside her or that he is crying a little in his heart. She has no idea that he is sad that she is gone for the day, sad that he did not feel wonder that day—a day that is now also gone.

That is why a father should never lose that wonder. He can remember that she is wonder-full. And he should never forget how precious his daughter is.

All daughters are precious, and have been since the beginning of time. A daughter named Helen of Troy was so precious that she caused the Trojan War when she was abducted by Paris, the Prince of Troy. While Helen was part of a Greek myth, there are certainly real-life examples of societies fighting for their women. There are men living today who will fight for their daughters.

Some Afghan men will fight to the death if someone steals a daughter. In 2002, I was meeting with an Afghan leader, a chief of one of two feuding clans, trying to convince him to call a truce. As we sat on the beautiful carpet spread out on the floor of his office, I asked him how all the shooting and feuding had begun. He explained rather matter-of-factly, through an interpreter, "They stole one of our women." Enough said in that part of the world.

Two of my young Afghan interpreters were working with us, risking their lives every day, mainly to earn money to afford a wife. Each needed between $3,000 and $5,000 for a good woman—closer to the higher number if she is pretty, can cook, and has all of her teeth. We might criticize many of their customs regarding women, but Afghan girls, by their definition, are precious.

In some other countries, women are not so precious. Parents actually abort countless fetuses when it is learned they are female. It is hard to believe, but they eliminate female fetuses because the fathers demand a male child. A man who would do that is feeling no wonder at all. The wonder is all gone. The men living in those wonder-less countries have gone full circle on the "How Men Perceive Women" cycle.

Girls are also precious because they love. They love their toys. And their friends. And their homes.

And they love their dads.

"Thank heaven for little girls, for little girls get bigger every day . . . no matter where no matter who, for without them, what would little boys do?"[2]

Most of the time, fathers love their daughters. But sadly, sometimes they don't do enough to protect their little girls. Dads often protect daughters less than they protect their car, house, or identity.

Why have I never heard of a Daughter-Theft Prevention company, despite the fact they are much more precious than an identity? I wonder if there are more girls being taken than identities around the world.

Governments fall and countries crumble when they do not protect their daughters. Entire civilizations fail when the men no longer feel wonder. Did the empires of Rome, Greece, or Persia really fail on the battlefield? No. They failed because their men no longer cherished little girls, their daughters, and they no longer felt wonder about their women. That is my theory.

> **"Having two daughters changed my perspective on a lot of things, and I definitely have a newfound respect for women. And I think I finally became a good and real man when I had a daughter."[3]**
>
> **—Mark Wahlberg**

Maybe that is one reason the Afghans have survived for thousands of years. Whatever people say about Afghans and their treatment of women (which is not good), Afghan men protect their women and will fight for them—to the death. And Afghan men don't take that lightly.

Dads, it is time to put down the wax and back away from the car.

Time to let go of the TV remote, the iPad, and the newspaper. It's time to remember that our girls are more precious than anything in life. They are more precious than our sports cars, our country, our identities, and life itself.

Parents, it is time to protect our girls. It is time to fight for them, to die for them, and to live for them.

And it's time to teach our daughter some spy skills. Let's turn her into Bond, Jane Bond.

NOTES

1. Victor Hugo, "A Ma Fille Adèle."

2. Alan Jay Lerner and Frederick Loewe, "Thank Heaven for Little Girls" (1957), sung by Maurice Chevalier, *Gigi,* 1958.

3. Mark Wahlberg, interview with Lori Berger, "He-man? Ha! Says Mark Wahlberg," redbookmag.com, February 1, 2012, http://www.redbookmag. com/love-sex/mens-perspective/interviews/a13429/mark-wahlberg-interview/.

3
How Men Target

"The serpent beguiled me, and I did eat."

—Genesis 3:13

A serpent "more subtle than any beast of the field," had tempted Eve, the first woman, to eat a piece of fruit through subtle persuasion. "Ye shall not surely die . . . ye shall be as gods," he argued (Genesis 3:4–5). Eve was deceived. The beguiling had begun.

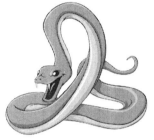

Now, thousands of years later, it continues. The sons of Adam are still subtle. And the daughters of Eve are not merely beguiled but are sometimes betrayed, befuddled, bluffed, burned, and bewildered. They are also seduced, exploited, duped, double-crossed, played, gamed, lured, conned, and cheated. Some men do it so subtly that it is now an art form: the art of manipulation.

Some sons of Adam have learned a lot over the thousands of years and are true artists. Unfortunately, the daughters of Eve are still talking to snakes.

Joe, a good friend and father of two teenage girls, once told me that he hates all young men, or snakes, as we still call them. He said that he hates them because he knows what they want, largely because Joe was once a young man and wanted the same thing. Now they want his daughters.

When I first heard Joe utter the word "hate," I found his comment a little harsh. *Don't be hatin'*, I thought. But now that my daughter has reached her teenage years and young men are targeting her as surely as

I hunted sources in the CIA, I find that I agree with Joe. I actually find myself "hatin'" young men too. (Yes, I said it.)

I was once a young snake, just like Joe. I used manipulation on my mother to get an extra cookie when I was young and on a young lady to get a kiss as a student in college. I then used manipulation on spies to steal secrets as a covert intelligence officer in the CIA. I was a manipulating snake.

As a covert operations officer in the CIA, I practiced the art of espionage. I do not consider espionage exactly satanic, but it is similar to what happened to Eve. It is the subtle art of manipulation. Spies, or operations officers, beguile and manipulate people for information. And I imagine that espionage continued after Adam and Eve were kicked out of the garden, when Eve sent one of her kids to go find out what Adam was doing in the garage.

While that first goal of manipulation—getting Eve to eat the fruit—has changed, the techniques are similar. Spying in today's world is carried out much as it always has been. It consists of pursuing someone—a target—based upon two basic criteria: access and vulnerabilities. The target must have both; if she is without one or the other, she is not worth pursuing.

ACCESS

This potential source must have access to what we want, which is intelligence. *Intelligence* is a fancy name for information that an intelligence-gathering agency like the CIA needs. The intelligence can be anything from how a country will vote at the next United Nations General Assembly to what its military is planning against us. The potential source must have access to that information, often needed for national security. The source must be able to provide the information through her position or contacts.

VULNERABILITIES

A potential source must also have weaknesses that will leave her susceptible to recruitment and manipulation. These vulnerabilities are personal flaws that render her susceptible to bribes or persuasion. There are many different types of vulnerabilities, from basic human appetite— "Hmm, I'm hungry, and that apple sure looks good"—to more complicated emotions: "I hate my boss," "I'm jealous of my coworker," or "I want a new car." Most vulnerabilities are in the form of intense emotions or desires. And they expose the target to recruitment, to one degree or another.

The vast majority of people do not have serious vulnerabilities and are therefore not recruitable, at least not most of the time. Hundreds of diplomats, businessmen, and military officers that I encountered were not vulnerable to my manipulation when I met them, at least not at that particular time in their life. Interestingly, an operations officer will sometimes place a target on the "back burner" until she becomes vulnerable at some future time. Operations officers are not just subtle; they are also patient.

A modern-day snake, or sexual predator, will target women in much the same way intelligence operatives target sources.

First, men look for women with access. In other words, they prefer women who can provide access to what they want. A football player on my college team boasted that his goal was to have sex with one hundred women before he graduated. That is extremely callous thinking. Another classmate confided, or boasted, that as a young man, he wanted to have sex with a woman from every country of the world. Just as callous.

I have to confess that I once thought I would try to kiss a different girl for every letter of the alphabet (Anne, Brenda, Cathy, and so on). Maybe this thinking was not quite as destructive, but it was just as manipulative and callous.

Some predators will also pursue women with vulnerabilities. They will search for women who are experiencing feelings of anger, heartache, or loneliness. Once a predator has detected a weakness, or combination of weaknesses, he will then try to exploit them to his benefit.

In 2014, I spoke to a group of young ladies at a girls' summer camp sponsored by my church, warning them that some men will assess them based upon whether they are an attractive target—a phrase used in both spy and romance terminology—and based on their vulnerabilities. I asked them if they could guess what vulnerabilities a target in espionage or romance could have in common. These young girls readily listed several: feelings of jealousy,

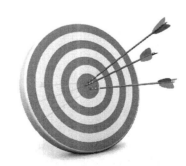

isolation, and sadness. They identified the same harmful human emotions that render young ladies vulnerable to a predator.

During the late 1980s, before I was married, I was dating a young woman in the Northern Virginia area. Her younger sister came to visit, partly because she had broken up (or was "terminated," in CIA terminology) with her boyfriend and was understandably heartbroken. She was also vulnerable. One evening, she returned to her sister's apartment in tears. When asked what had happened, she revealed that an older man, a coworker of her sister's, had tried to take advantage of her vulnerability.

He had invited her into a bedroom, where he comforted her, consoled her, told her that she was beautiful, and called her ex-boyfriend a fool. He said all this while rubbing her shoulders and her back, slowly easing her down to a prone position, where he tried to kiss her. An intelligence agency would have been proud of his technique, if not for the fact that she had no access to foreign intelligence . . . and that she was underage.

Unfortunately, along with "sugar and spice and everything nice" comes a trustful nature. Actually, most of us, particularly the youth, do not anticipate evil. And this young lady never dreamed that a well-dressed professional would try to exploit her pain. She never saw it coming. This is why snakes prefer to be subtle in their efforts.

Many sexual predators are not so subtle when their goals are not met. They become frustrated, aggressive, and even angry. My wife informed me that the above scenario happens to every woman at one time or another. She had two relatives who tried to sexually assault her during her youth in Africa. Both were men she trusted—men she treated with respect. One offered her a ride home but detoured to his factory to show her where he worked. Once there, he tried several manipulative tactics, including bribery—offering to give her mother financial support—and then force. She was forced to fight him off. The second man tried more stealthily: watching her and offering gifts, compliments, and feigned kindness. He spun a web as deftly as a spider for months. Again, she trusted, never dreaming that he would be manipulative. He asked if she would accompany him to his office to retrieve some money. When they arrived, he locked the door and assaulted her. She again had to fight.

She was lucky that her father had warned her about those types of men and what they would be after—her. In his naïveté, however, he did not know that she would be attacked by men in her own extended family, so he did not prepare her for assaults from her own relatives.

Interestingly, the CIA teaches its officers to be aware of potential blowback if an approach, or pitch, is rejected by the target. Blowback, or negative consequences, in the CIA might include being imprisoned or being beaten by the local police. If he is lucky, an intelligence officer will only be labeled *persona non grata*, ("an unwelcome person" in diplomatic terms) and deported back to the United States. Blowback in espionage, in any form, is a constant concern.

Once while pursuing a "hard target" (from a rogue country like Iran or North Korea), I invited him to a restaurant for lunch. During the lunch, I began to let him know who I really was and what I really wanted—which was to recruit him to work for the CIA, and not just to be great friends and enjoy Parisian pastries together. I could almost see the light bulb illuminate above his head when he realized my true intentions. I then saw an expression of anger replace the light bulb. He jumped to his feet and told me, rather loudly, "You have chosen the wrong target!"

Oops. That is one form of blowback. I quickly reassured him that he must have misunderstood me, that I had no intentions of targeting him and that I actually did enjoy sharing Parisian pastries with him, and I backpedaled as best I could. Blowback happens in the spy world.

In romantic targeting, similar scenarios play themselves out every evening in nightclubs, hotels, convention halls, business offices, and schools. Unfortunately, there seems to be little risk of blowback for predators who target young women. Women often just join a "secret society of abuse" rather than expose the predator.

They decide to suffer in silence. According to a study by the Department of Justice, published on December 11, 2014, only 20 percent of victims of sexual assault on college campuses ever report it.[1] The study also found that for both college students and nonstudents, "the offender was known to the victim in about 80% of rape and sexual assault victimizations." That is an interesting but sad correlation: 80 percent of women who are assaulted do not report it, and 80 percent of them knew their attacker.

My wife did not report either of the men who assaulted her. She was probably more embarrassed than they were, which seems to be the case in many situations. Young women often think it is better to "sweep it under the rug" and try to forget about it. Maybe she will just avoid the overly aggressive athlete on campus. Or she will decline future rides home from the creepy cousin. Anything rather than tell someone about it. I think sexual predators deserve some negative consequences. They deserve some blowback.

RECRUITMENT CYCLE

When targeting a source, an operations officer will try to move a relationship through a recruitment cycle (another cycle!). This is the "bread and butter" of espionage, which consists of five steps:

1. Spot: identify a target.
2. Assess: determine her access and vulnerabilities.
3. Develop: build rapport and trust.
4. Recruit: enlist her as an asset/source.
5. Terminate: cut off the relationship.

It is striking how a guy with bad intentions (GWBI—let's call him a Gweebi), routinely follows similar steps of the recruitment cycle when targeting a young woman. A Gweebi will look to spot a young woman, assess her for vulnerabilities, develop trust and rapport, and then recruit her (or seduce her). He will then "terminate" her when she is of no further use. A Gweebi follows almost an identical recruitment cycle as a covert operations officer. He is careful, subtle, and often methodical. Gweebis can be premeditated predators—or sexual operations officers.

While in college, I was dating a young lady with an older sister who was probably twenty or twenty-one years of age—a beautiful young woman. I met the sister when she returned from the same university we were attending. Unfortunately, she was heartbroken at the treatment she had received from some of the young men at the school. She was a striking blonde and had obviously received a great deal of attention, some of it unwelcome.

When she returned home that summer, a much older man—an owner of a local car dealership—noticed her (*spotting*) at a club and introduced himself. His attention was also unwanted, but he persisted (*assessing*) and eventually offered her a car from his lot, free of charge (*developing*). She resisted, but he persuaded her to take one of his vehicles back to school after summer break. She unwisely accepted his offer. At the end of the semester, she returned home with the car.

She did not yet agree to date him, but he saw her from time to time, and he offered her another even nicer vehicle (more *developing*). She again accepted his offer and drove it back to school, with no strings attached.

As it turned out, there were strings, namely her feelings of obligation—most likely that she must owe him something for his kindness. How kind he was to lend her beautiful cars to take to school! He reeled her in as skillfully as a professional fisherman, using expensive, luxurious vehicles as bait.

When they eventually began to openly date, as she would call it, she felt obliged to introduce the car dealer to her father. The car dealer—more like car loaner—was not keen on the idea, probably because he was actually a few years older than her father, but he eventually relented. I can only imagine how that meeting went over.

A year later, my girlfriend and I went to visit her car-borrowing sister, who was now living with her older boyfriend. When we knocked, she appeared at the door, a changed woman (*recruitment*). I hardly recognized her. She had completely transformed into a pliable, obedient, live-in mistress. She now wore her hair up in a bun and sported a light blue, one-piece jump-suit, complete with a broach—an outfit that you might expect to see on a much older woman. She was still attractive, but she looked much more his age at that point.

It bothered me to see her again, now a pliant captive. On the positive side, she will have all the luxury vehicles she could ever wish for, unless he has traded her in (the last step—*termination*) for a newer model.

That is how a man—a predatory man—will target a woman. It might not be simple to notice if he is being subtle, but it is possible to recognize and avoid his plan, if a woman is aware and if she uses her spy skills.

Is he moving you along the recruitment cycle?

1. Spot
2. Assess
3. Develop
4. Recruit
5. Terminate

NOTES

1. Lynn Langton and Sofi Sinozich, "Rape and Sexual Assault Victimization Among College-Age Females, 1995–2013," US Department of Justice, Bureau of Justice Statistics, December 2014.

4

How Men Influence

Although he probably considered himself very clever, the car dealer Casanova (of the previous chapter) was merely using one of the techniques identified by Professor Robert Cialdini in his 1984 book, *Influence: The Psychology of Persuasion*. Professor Cialdini's principles are largely based on his experiences with and studies of "compliance professionals": salespeople, fundraisers, recruiters, and so on. I would argue that sexual predators are seeking to be included in that group. It is interesting that their techniques seem so similar.

The following is a summary of Professor Cialdini's six principles—reciprocity, commitment, social proof, liking, authority, and scarcity[1]:

1. Reciprocity. Humans feel the need to "return favors, pay back debts, and treat others as they treat us."[2] This can lead a target to feel obliged to comply with another's wishes or to compromise and sacrifice her own intentions out of a desire to return the favor. Sound familiar? The car dealer (in the previous chapter) provided flashy cars to the young college girl in order to make her feel indebted.

Caution! Before accepting a date or a gift from a young man, ask yourself if you will feel obliged to reciprocate (possibly in the form of sexual favors or affection). A predatory man will often consider dinner and a movie simply to be a down payment on what he expects from a woman later in the evening. While a woman may be tempted to accept a "pity" date because she feels kindhearted or doesn't want to hurt the man's feelings by saying no, she should keep in mind that it is better to turn down the date or gift than feel indebted and unduly influenced later on. We'll discuss the dangers of a "pity" date in a later chapter.

2. Commitment (and consistency). Cialdini noted that we all "have a deep desire to be consistent."[3] For example, if a young lady has already shown some interest, dated, or invested in a relationship, she can feel compelled to continue or maintain that commitment. A clever, manipulative young man might even remind her of that fact: "We have been dating for a long time, we owe it to ourselves to see where the relationship goes."

Caution! Before continuing in a relationship, or deepening a commitment to someone, a young woman needs to ask herself if she will feel so "invested in this new course of action that (she) won't want to change (her) mind." In my opinion, women care much more about commitment than men, and they will sometimes try to preserve this investment in a relationship, even when the man is wrong for her.

There is no downside to developing a relationship slowly and carefully. Do not let yourself be bound by commitment to someone you do not yet know well. Treat a relationship a little like a gym membership: pay month to month, and do not sign up for a full year until you know what you are getting yourself into. There is a downside to being tied down to the wrong person. As England Dan and John Ford Coley sang, "Oh, how sad to belong to someone else when the right one comes along."[4]

3. Social proof. This is a need to "go along with the crowd." I find it interesting that a door-to-door salesman will note to me that several neighbors bought his product, hoping that I will feel the need to go along. *Heck,* we think. *It must be a great alarm system if the Jones family next door bought it!* Professor Cialdini notes, "We're particularly susceptible to this principle when we're feeling uncertain."[5]

Caution! A young lady might think, "Brittany and Bruce have been dating for such a long time, and they are so happy. I need to have a boyfriend too. I don't want to be the only girl without a boyfriend." Ladies, avoid the "herd mentality"! It's okay to be a third-wheel from time to time. And enjoy the calm and serenity of a drama-free life!

4. Liking. This is a rather obvious principle: we are more likely to be influenced by people that are likable. Professor Cialdini notes, "Likability comes in many forms—people might be similar or familiar to us, they might give us compliments, or we may just simply trust them."[6]

Caution! A young man who pursues a young woman might be from the same town, the same high school, or in the same club. So what? She needs to ask herself if she is dating someone because she has known him since sixth grade or because he is nice or because their parents are best friends. This might sound odd, but do not let likability cloud your judgment. Likability is not chemistry.

5. Authority. As a society, we are taught to respect and look up to people in authority. "Job titles, uniforms, and even accessories like cars or gadgets can lend an air of authority, and can persuade (a young woman) to accept what these people say."[7] That's why some men refer to their cars as "chick magnets." A car gives them an air of authority and is often merely bait to target, attract, or influence young, impressionable women. Positions of authority also give some men—from comedians to presidents—undue influence.

In the world of espionage there is a class of spies, or assets, called "agents of influence." This type of agent is recruited and then called upon to influence policy and decisions made by his government. Obviously, the higher the agent's rank or position in his government, the greater his ability to influence the government's policy decisions.

Unfortunately, as in espionage, the greater the authority enjoyed by a predator, the more influence he is able to wield over his target. A high-ranking commander in the military, a studio director, or a president can often exert much more pressure and influence over subordinates and victims.

Caution! Ladies, beware of overly friendly bosses, superiors in the military, or teachers. Remind yourself that respect for authority ends at the office or classroom. Respect the military, sure, but do not fall for a uniform. And do not let men who tell you they hold the keys to your career drive you and your career aspirations. Keep the keys to your ambition in your own hands.

6. Scarcity. Professor Cialdini writes that this principle "says that things are attractive when their availability is limited, or when we stand to lose the opportunity to acquire them on favorable terms."[8] Salesmen use this technique all the time: "Limited time offer!" Whenever I hear this line, I usually ask myself, "What? They won't make more?!"

Caution! A scarce, unique man—the new guy at school, the captain of the football team, the foreign exchange student—can have unreasonable, disproportionate influence over a young women because he is a "limited supply" item. He can use that influence to push a girl to do more than she would, or should, such as enter into a sexual relationship.

This summary of Cialdini's six principles ends with a warning: "Be careful how you use the six principles—it is easy to use them to mislead or deceive people—for instance, to sell products at unfair prices, or to exert undue influence."[9] Influence is a double-edged sword. I am actually trying to influence young women with this book: to influence them to be careful and to take steps to protect themselves. I hope that this book will be an influence for good in young women's lives.

But there are those out there who are trying, working, to be an influence for evil in women's lives. Young men: if you are reading this, even after I told you this book is not for you, do not try to exert influence over young women, or manipulate and exploit them. That is harmful, destructive behavior, and it would make you a predator.

I wonder if some men, especially predators, will consider me a traitor to the male gender for revealing how men attempt to influence women. After all, I am giving up the team's "playbook" on how men manipulate women. Truthfully, I do not feel like I have switched teams. I prefer to think of it as my having merely switched from offense to defense.

Is your date trying to exert influence through . . .

1. Reciprocity? *His paying for dinner and a movie is not a down payment for passion.*

2. Commitment? *Do not feel pressured to continue dating someone just because he has been your boyfriend or your friends have "coupled" you up. You do not belong to anyone.*

3. Social Proof? *Be free! Do not give in to peer pressure to be in a relationship.*

4. Liking? *Okay, it's nice that he's nice. So what? You want more than that.*

5. Authority? *Respect for authority ends when inappropriate behavior begins.*

6. Scarcity? *There are plenty of fish in the sea.*

NOTES

1. Robert Cialdini, *Influence: The Psychology of Persuasion* (New York: Harper Business, 1984).

2. Keith Jackson, "Cialdini's Six Principles of Influence: Convincing Others to Say 'Yes,'" accessed September 3, 2015, http://www.mindtools.com/pages/article/six-principles-influence.htm.

3. Ibid.

4. England Dan and John Ford Coley, "Sad to Belong," May 1977.

5. Keith Jackson, "Cialdini's Six Principles of Influence."

6. Ibid.

7. Ibid.

8. Ibid.

9. Ibid.

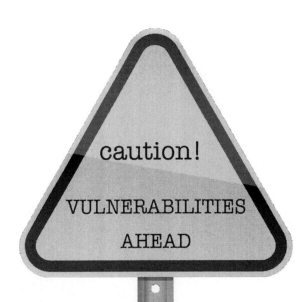

5

Vulnerabilities

**"Men think about women.
Women think about what men
think about them."**[1]

—Peter Ustinov

Some women find themselves vulnerable from time to time. It happens. No one can walk through the minefields of high school, college, or the workplace without stepping on hidden, sometimes volatile, feelings of anger, fear, jealousy, or loneliness. All of these emotions happen to each one of us. These emotions are part of the human experience.

What matters most is that ladies recognize when they are feeling these emotions, know when they are vulnerable, and avoid situations where they may be manipulated. A woman needs to know *when* she is feeling these emotional vulnerabilities, *where* she is feeling them, and *with whom*.

Even CIA officers are vulnerable at one time or another. That said, not many are like Harold Nicholson, who betrayed his country for $300,000 cash from the Russians and who is now serving a life sentence for treason in a federal "super-max" prison, in Colorado. Very few follow the path of former operations officer Aldrich Ames, who betrayed his country for a Jaguar, a new house, and whatever luxuries he enjoyed before he was arrested. After his conviction, he claimed that he had "his reasons" for committing treason. Authorities reportedly found more than fifty purses and five hundred pairs of shoes in his home when he was arrested. I doubt that his reasons, or shoes, were worth a life sentence in a super-max. And I doubt he is having a super-good life.

How many CIA officers are lucky enough to just not be vulnerable at the wrong place and wrong time? How many have been lucky enough to not encounter a Russian intelligence officer at a cocktail party on the same night they were fighting with a wife or the same day they were passed over for promotion or when they were thousands of dollars in debt or were falling down drunk? Maybe many were lucky that they were not vulnerable in the wrong place at the wrong time with the wrong person.

So first and foremost, a young woman needs to protect herself, from herself. She needs to guard against her own weaknesses. Let's talk about vulnerabilities. There are all types and degrees of weaknesses, as varied as there are young women:

1. Vanity. Young ladies can feel unattractive and unwanted at the wrong place and wrong time (WPWT). In today's culture, girls are bombarded with images of what is considered beautiful. Media floods all of us with images of ideal women, models and actors, and even specific body parts on a daily basis. Girls are programmed to want to be like them.

> **"The rarest thing in the world is a woman who is pleased with photographs of herself."[2]**
>
> **—Elizabeth Metcalf**

And young men are programmed to want those women with those body parts. These boys then target girls who are willing to advertise their matching body parts. The girls are then hunted by the programmed boys and bask in that short-term attention.

Young women who do not have the ideal figure can feel unwanted. So they either convince their dads to purchase them new body parts from a cosmetic surgeon in order to join the other girls who are exploited by the programmed boys, or they decide to wear more revealing clothes to gain attention and then be exploited by the programmed boys.

Ladies, resist the programming and the brainwashing. Learn to distinguish between reality and perception. Real life is not photoshopped, airbrushed, or enhanced. It sounds cliché, but just be yourself. And choose to be content with yourself.

2. Jealousy. Ladies can feel jealousy at the WPWT. My teenage daughter told me that she can even feel jealous while watching a movie of a young actress who is dating a seemingly "perfect" young man. She will find herself wishing that she were the girlfriend in that "perfect" relationship.

But young ladies often do not see the whole story. They do not see the handsome young actor as he enters drug rehabilitation after filming, or see his mug shot when he is arrested for punching his mother. She only sees the airbrushed, photoshopped image, which is an illusion that can make anyone jealous.

Magazines, movies, and music videos all manipulate women, especially the tastes and perception of women. Jealous girls then feel that if they dress a certain way or act a certain way, they will have that boyfriend and that romance, complete with a romantic drive through the country, accompanied by Academy Award–winning music, costumes, and cinematography.

Jealousy breeds resentment and desperation, both of which can lead to bad choices with bad men. Jealousy will lead a woman to do things that she would not otherwise do in a relationship with a man whom she would not otherwise even consider dating.

3. Curiosity. Ladies can feel curious at the WPWT. Curiosity is a powerful, motivational emotion. CIA officers can even recruit sources based on their curiosity. A target of mine (I still feel guilty referring to people as targets, but that is the reality of the spy world) agreed to meet with me based solely on his curiosity. He just wanted to meet a real-life CIA officer. He had seen me at cocktail parties and diplomatic functions around town and had wondered if I was a spy. He was curious to see what it was like to meet with the CIA, and he put himself at risk because of it.

> **"To awake a woman's curiosity is to make her pliable."[3]**
>
> **—Reverend William Scott Downey**

Women seem to be especially curious. And curiosity can be a good thing, especially in the sciences, mathematics, and other school subjects, where she can learn about gravity, botany, chemistry, aviation, ceramics, music, and more. It is curiosity that drives us to learn.

But curiosity in a social life or the world of romance can be a vulnerability. Sadly, sexual predators know this and will often make great efforts to appeal to a woman's curiosity, first to attract her attention, and then to manipulate her once he has her close to him.

Curiosity can lead a young woman to be willing to try more—to do more—than she should with young men, especially strangers. Curiosity can lead her to watch more pornographic or violent movies, to drink more, to try drugs and then harder drugs, and to be more immoral. Once she is hooked by curiosity, she can be manipulated to sacrifice what she holds dear. She might forget who she is and what she stands for.

4. Anger. A young woman can feel anger at the WPWT. A friend once boasted that she had married her husband because she was angry with her father. She felt that her father was too controlling by not accepting her boyfriend, and she resented that her father would not treat her as an adult. So she decided to "show" him by marrying her fiancé when she was still very young and he much older.

It turned out that her father was right about the guy. Her husband turned out to be a man with several personal problems, including heavy drinking, drug addiction, and criminal behavior. After several years, and three children, he died of a drug overdose.

Anger causes excessive drinking, fights, road rage, resentment, thoughts of revenge, and even murder. How many prisoners are incarcerated because of their anger? How many spies, or traitors, were recruited based upon anger: that she wasn't paid enough, that she did not receive a choice work assignment, that a boyfriend dumped her for another? Anger blurs and blinds our judgment to the point that we no longer see the mines in a social minefield or even care that they are there. Recognize when you are angry, and either cool off or be careful.

5. Arrogance. Ladies can feel arrogant at the WPWT. Ladies that put "me, myself, and I" before everyone and everything render themselves vulnerable. Arrogance, or pride, is actually the most sought-after weakness by operations officers in espionage. It is the greatest vulnerability.

After twenty-three years of "hunting" humans for intelligence, I grew skilled at identifying the arrogant ones. I could almost smell arrogance, and still can. I wonder if it is arrogant of me to say that I can detect arrogance.

A religious leader once said, "Pride is a deadly cancer. It is a gateway sin that leads to a host of other human weaknesses."[4] Arrogance does lead to a lot of sin, or bad choices, whatever you want to call it. Arrogance—this me-first attitude—can lead to crimes as innocuous as jaywalking and graffiti to more serious offenses like embezzlement, burglary, rape, assault, and even treason. Aldrich Ames was arrogant, which lead him to a feeling of entitlement and greed and then more arrogance that he would not get caught. Arrogance led him to feel invincible when, in actuality, it turned him into a target, a soft target, for the Russians.

Arrogance in women can lead to immodesty and immorality (both old-fashioned words in today's society, it seems), and it can turn a young woman into a soft target for predators. A predator can spot, or smell, an overly inflated ego as skillfully as any operations officer.

Be confident but not arrogant. Find the line between the two, and do not cross it.

6. Greed. Traitors are often motivated by greed. I recruited and handled many sources based upon their uncontrollable desire for money. Young women can feel this same hunger, or longing for more, at the WPWT. Greed, which is really a byproduct of arrogance, causes people to want, to want more, and then to want more at all cost.

At school I read a play called *Antigone* by French writer Jean Anouilh. During one scene, Creon tells Antigone, "Life flows like water, and you young people let it run away through your fingers. Shut your hands; hold on to it."[6] Some people who seek too much in life—who feel greed—end up wanting too much, and will attempt to live life with their fingers open and spread out rather than cupping them together and cherishing what they have. They are not satisfied with enough; they demand more. How much better it is to cup our fingers, to take what we can, be satisfied with enough life to quench our thirst, and enjoy it!

> **A man approaches a young lady and asks, "Would you sleep with me for one million dollars?"**
>
> **"Yes," she quickly replies.**
>
> **"Okay, how about twenty dollars."**
>
> **"Of course not! What do you think I am?" she shoots back.**
>
> **"We have already established what you are," he answered. "We are now just haggling over the price."[5]**

An interesting study by BYU Professor Stanley Taylor and a graduate student in 1998 researched the motivations people have to become spies and betray their country.[7] The study concluded that during World War II and the early Cold War, motivation was primarily ideological, but greed began to take over during the 1960s. Professor Taylor noted, "We observed the changing nature, the changing motivation of American traitors." He added, "I suspect, too, that society has just become more materialistic."

Greed causes men to try and have sexual relations with one hundred women. And greed causes women to want to be included in that secret, sorrowful club. Greed is why some are living in a super-max prison and others in super-max heartache.

Learn to cup your fingers to drink in enough happiness and enough life. Be happy with enough and avoid cravings for more.

7. Despair. Girls can feel hopeless at the WPWT with the wrong person (WP). In places where poverty is rampant, like Africa, people are often mired in hopelessness. Feelings of hopelessness, or helplessness, lead to desperation. Desperation then leads a young lady to a weakness: to sacrifice herself, her pride, and her virtue, hoping to buy a future. Countless mistresses around the world are manipulated by rich old men that prey upon their desperation, brought on by hopelessness (funny thing, I've never seen a beautiful young woman with a *poor* old man).

If a young lady loses hope, the antidote is to look for someone to help her find it. I worked as a job coach for several years after I retired. Some of my clients with disabilities would express hopelessness at not finding a job, at being alienated from society, or at being criticized for their inabilities. I regularly told them to ignore those people who would drag them down and to listen to those who would elevate them.

A young lady who lacks hope can choose whom to listen to. Hopefully her family, friends, teachers, and religious leaders are all trying to build her up rather than tear her down. If not, she can find associates who will. She can listen to those who tell her that she is a wonderful girl with potential and a future. She can choose to believe the affirming influences in her life. She can choose to think positive.

I often think about Will Rhea Winfrey when I feel despair. Will Rhea was a teammate and good friend of my father's from his football team of the late 1930s and also a fellow WWII veteran. After the war, Will Rhea returned home and married his sweetheart but soon suffered a devastating loss: he lost his eyesight. Years later, he suffered another tragedy: losing his wife in an automobile accident. When he was in his nineties, he ended up living in the woods near Somerville, Tennessee, all by himself. His relatives checked in on him frequently, but he mostly managed for himself.

Will Rhea was always so upbeat when we spoke on the phone that I just had to meet him in person. So when I retired, my family and I drove through his town and stayed with him for a couple of days on our way west. I had the chance to ask him how he managed to stay so positive after all the adversity in his life. He told me, in his wonderful Southern drawl, "Well, any day that I can wake up and put my two feet on the floor is a good day."

Lack of hope is a vulnerability. Never lose hope. Choose hope!

8. Loneliness. Girls can feel lonely at the WPWTWP. *Psychology Today* quotes Dr. Jill P. Weber, who wrote:

> [A woman's] social awareness is a tremendous strength and when properly developed through the years can be used beneficially in adult life. However, caring can become a trap when a woman becomes so committed to staying connected to others that she loses touch with her separate sense of self. At the extreme, self-esteem may come to depend almost completely on relationships with others—for example, if they have a socially packed weekend they feel great about themselves—if they are alone with time to fill, suddenly they feel like they have done something wrong.
>
> In this type of situation, a woman comes to fear being alone and works to avoid that circumstance at all cost. This can include the crippling effect of "friends" or romantic partners who do not care about her needs. Having a warm body to fill the space becomes more important than how that "warm body" actually treats and relates to her. . . .
>
> When it comes to romance, women in this situation may find themselves in a revolving door, where romantic partners enter and exit their lives quickly. Not wishing to be alone, the woman may work overtime to play a role that she believes will make her acceptable. Playing a role in order to please someone else takes her further away from knowing and accepting her true self.[8]

We all know the woman who cannot seem to last for more than a few days between boyfriends or without an admirer or so-called love. Sexual predators look for her. They look for the woman who is feeling lonely, especially when she is "on the rebound." These men see lonely women as easy pickings—easy to pick up and easy to take advantage of. In short, these women who have just ended a relationship, or a marriage, are vulnerable.

If you find yourself feeling lonely, call a friend or a family member. Surround yourself with good people. There is safety in numbers.

9. Overly tolerant. Women can feel too tolerant at the WPWTWP. This might rub some people the wrong way since tolerance seems to go hand-in-hand with our current climate of political correctness. But just because bigots are intolerant does not mean that the rest of us should be tolerant of everything. Should a woman tolerate an insensitive or rude boyfriend? Should she ever tolerate physical or emotional abuse? Should she tolerate immorality, disloyalty, or dishonesty? Should she tolerate unruly nose hairs, or hairy ears? My wife doesn't.

Too much tolerance can be a vulnerability. Women can be so tolerant that they surrender to a jerk's insistence to go on a date. She might already know that he is not right for her—that he is mean or rude—but she tolerates his behavior just the same because she does not want to appear judgmental to him or others in her circle of friends.

> **"Vice is a monster of so frightful mien, that to be feared needs but to be seen. But seen too oft, familiar with her face, first we pity, then endure, then embrace."[9]**
>
> **—Alexander Pope**

She might consider it intolerant of her to decline an invitation from a criminal or a liar just because he is a foreigner or is of a different race, religion, or state. So rather than be called judgmental or intolerant, a young woman will date a bully, a drunk, or any young man who has more faults than qualities. And she might even marry him and invest years of her life until he cheats on her with a younger woman he met at the gym. Tolerance can cost her a lot.

Being from out-of-state is not a reason to reject him, nor should it be a pass for his misbehavior. Be picky. Be a little intolerant.

10. Overly compassionate. A young woman can feel too much compassion, at the WPWTWP. This might seem like another odd vulnerability on my list. But I believe that women sometimes feel almost an instinctive, motherly urge to fix men. Maybe that's a reason why some women gravitate toward "fixer-upper" men.

I believe that women are nurturing and compassionate by nature. Women may feel compelled to help a young man overcome problems with alcohol, drugs, or violent tendencies. But this nurturing spirit, this compassionate attitude (maybe a little curiosity again?) can cause her to sacrifice too much, even her life.

> **"A kind heart he hath: a woman would run through fire and water for such a kind heart."[10]**
>
> **—William Shakespeare**

During a life-saving class at the swimming pool, we were taught to guard our own life before attempting to save a drowning person: first try to reach out to a drowning person with a long pole or ladder, or throw him a rope, life jacket, or seat cushion. Even row a boat to reach him. But the choice of last resort is to dive into the water because a drowning victim will often grab the rescuer, and even climb on top of her, to keep his head above water. Many would-be rescuers end up drowning along with the victim.

Ladies, throw a young man some help, but do not sacrifice yourself by diving into a relationship based on pity or compassion. Do not allow yourself to be pulled under by someone with troubles enough to drown you both.

And since women are inherently compassionate, they can be suckers for compassion, or perceived kindness, when they see it. Young women can be manipulated by gestures of kindness that might be merely another "down payment" by the predator to get what he wants (much like dinner and a movie).

Sometimes, it's genuine kindness from a nice young man and sometimes it's not. That's what a young lady has to find out. She must find out why he is offering to buy dinner. Why is he offering to take her home? Why is he offering to buy her jewelry? Why is he offering her a car for the semester? What exactly are his intentions?

I hope that every young woman will be aware of her own weaknesses and recognize when she feels them. She can then avoid being vulnerable, or at least showing vulnerability at the wrong place (Internet, gym, nightclub, sorority house) at the wrong time (late at night, after work, when she is tired) and to the wrong person (fools, stalkers, sexual predators, or worse).

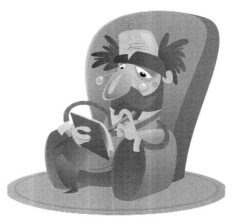

To protect herself, a woman needs to be first and foremost self-aware: aware of her emotions, weaknesses, insecurities, and vulnerabilities, and where she is feeling them. Self-awareness is the first step in her self-defense.

So analyze yourself like a psychologist. Be your own Dr. Phil!

Realize when you feel . . .

1. Vanity
2. Jealousy
3. Curiosity
4. Anger
5. Arrogance
6. Greed
7. Despair
8. Loneliness
9. Overly tolerant
10. Overly compassionate

NOTES

1. Michael Powell, *The Mamouth Book of Great British Humour* (London: Robinson, 2010).

2. M. P. Singh, *Quote Unquote* (Chichester: Lotus Books, 2006), 296.

3. William Scott Downey, *Downey's Proverbs* (Boston: E. Walker, 1858), 30.

4. Dieter F. Uchtdorf, "Pride and the Priesthood" *Ensign*, October 2010.

5. Old joke, unknown source.

6. Jean Anouilh, *Antigone: A Tragedy*, translated by Lewis Galantière (New York: Random House, 1946), 41.

7. Kim Howey, *BYU Magazine*, Summer 1998.

8. Jill P. Weber "When You Can't Stand Being Alone with Yourself," *Psychology Today*, November 19, 2013.

9. Alexander Pope, "Essay on Man Epistle III," Poetry Foundation, accessed August 9, 2015, http://www.poetryfoundation.org/poem/174166.

10. William Shakespeare, "Merry Wives of Windsor," *The Oxford Shakespeare: The Complete Works* (Oxford: Oxford University, 2005).

6
Vetting

Near the end of the film *Avatar*, the female Na'vi Neytiri sees Jake Sully for the first time in his weak, human body. As she holds him, they both look into each other's eyes and say, "I see you."[1] She sees him for who he really is. She sees more than a disabled human; she sees who he really is inside, and she sees him for who he can become.

I have told many young ladies, including my daughter, that a girl should see a boy at his worst: when he is hot, tired, thirsty, hungry, angry, upset, frustrated, and maybe all those emotions at the same time. And she needs to see him when he is vulnerable. She should see a young man after his team loses a basketball game, when he is in a hurry and his mother asks him to take out the garbage, when his little sister needs him but he is playing video games with friends, when his car runs out of gas on the way to work, or when he hits his thumb with a hammer.

> *"Il est tres simple: l'essential est invisible pour les yeux . . . on ne voit bien qu'avec le coeur."*[2] (Trans. "It is very simple; the essential is invisible to the eye. We can only see well with our hearts.") —*The Little Prince*

How do we tell the good from the bad? That's often what it boils down to in life. How to tell a good mango from a bad one before we eat one and have short-term, painful stomachaches? How to tell a good guy from a bad before a girl dates him or marries him and suffers long-term, painful heartache? The best way to tell a good man from a bad is by vetting.

Vetting means to carefully, critically examine someone—to truly come to know who that person is, what he aspires to be, what he wishes for, how he sees and treats others, and what he wants out of life. To vet someone is to dissect him, figuratively, like the frog in your science class. It is used to probe inside him, to see inside his heart, his head, and right down to his soul.

A little vetting can go a long way. A little vetting can save a lady an awful lot. Imagine what could be prevented by simple vetting of a potential boyfriend: wasted efforts, emotions, lives, money, and years of suffering. Vetting can help avoid the lost years—years that a young lady could have spent dating real men, good men.

I know that I will vet every young man who wants to have any kind of relationship with my daughter because I want my daughter to find a great young man. And because I do not think that anyone should hate ignorantly. I prefer to vet a young man so I can hate him intelligently, accurately, and rationally!

In espionage, vetting is a constant procedure that is done before recruitment of a source, after recruitment, and throughout the life of the operation until the source is terminated. When a covert officer neglects vetting a source, she does it at her own peril because a source can be friendly one day and a foe the next when he is *bought* and *turned* (turned into a double agent) by another country. One day the source is giving us intelligence, the next he is giving it to someone else.

Many people in our society are for "rent," even boyfriends. Ladies rent them for an evening, a few dates, or for a month or for two, but do not really own them. I believe that young men can be *turned* as easily as an agent. Girls should consider a man unvetted, or untested, until marriage, and even then she should continue to keep an eye on him.

In the spy world, an operations officer will vet someone for authenticity, reliability, truthfulness, and hostile control (being controlled by another intelligence organization). She must know if her source is really who he says he is, whether she can depend on the source or not, and if he will be somewhere when she wants him to be there, exactly where she wants him, acting the way he should act. She wants to know if he always tells the truth. And last, she needs to know whether he is being controlled by someone or something else. Could he be a double agent?

Some people might mistakenly believe that the CIA might not really care so much if a source has all of the above qualities as long as he has information to give. This is wrong. After all, the intelligence officer's life is often in the source's hands, and vice versa.

Vetting in our everyday life and in romantic espionage is just as important. It is equally crucial that young women vet boyfriends for the same qualities. And she needs to vet him with blinders on—that is to say—without regard for how hot, handsome, rich, or smart the young man is. She should vet a young man as if her life depends upon it. Because it often does.

Would Susan Powell, the young mother believed to have been murdered by her husband, still be alive if she had carefully vetted and examined her future husband—for truthfulness, anger issues, reliability, or sanity? Would her two young boys, whom her husband subsequently murdered in a fire, still be alive?

Would Nicole Brown Simpson still be alive if she, or her parents, had carefully and critically vetted her future husband, the handsome O. J. Simpson—for unfettered arrogance, jealousy, or uncontrollable anger?

Young ladies are not the only ones who should vet a potential suitor. Parents should vet a man as if their daughter's life depends upon it. How much vetting did the parents of Elizabeth Smart conduct when they first gave money to a homeless man, and then invited him home and introduced him to their children? Brian Mitchell, or "Emmanuel" (as he called himself), a self-described Jesus and a psychopath, later told a captive Elizabeth that he had began preparing to snatch her from the moment he saw her, an entire year before he kidnapped and repeatedly raped her.

When we neglect vetting a young man who is becoming involved with our daughter, we do it at our own peril.

1. Vet him for authenticity. Is he who he says he is? Does he really work where he says he does? Does he actually go to the university that he claims to attend? Mark Hacking, a student at the University of Utah, murdered his wife, Lori, on July 19, 2004. Lori had planned to move to North Carolina with her husband, where he claimed he would attend the University of North Caroline-Chapel Hill medical school. A police investigation of Hacking revealed that he had not completed an undergraduate degree at the University of Utah, and that his intended medical school had no record of him ever having applied. Hacking first lied to his wife about his schooling. He then murdered her when she found out the truth too late. Hacking pleaded guilty to Lori's murder and is in prison.

I am only slightly embarrassed to admit that I called my future daughter-in-law at her claimed workplace a few months prior to her marriage to my son, as a test. The operator answered and connected me. I had a pretext for calling—asking a few questions about the upcoming marriage—and soon ended the telephone call, feeling a little guilty. But I successfully found out that she was an authentic, bona fide employee at that company. She passed the test.

I was not always so suspicious. In my mid-twenties I met a Venezuelan woman at a singles' church dance. Over the next few weeks, we became friends, but fortunately, as it turned out, not romantically involved. As we grew acquainted, she claimed that she was a member of my church, that she was attending Georgetown University, that she was from a wealthy Venezuelan family involved in the oil business, and that she owned a nice BMW. She also told me that she was suffering from a brain tumor and was being treated at a local hospital. (Yep, I believed all that.)

One day, I went to pick her up at her home in Georgetown, after she had claimed that her vehicle was damaged in an accident. Interestingly, and suspiciously, this was the first time I had been to her home because she always insisted on meeting me in various places around town.

I knocked on the door, and a woman and small child appeared. I asked for Estella and the woman replied that she was not home. I then remarked, innocently, that Estella's BMW looked fine after the accident. "What accident?" replied the rather startled woman as she glanced at the car in the garage. "That is my car, and it has not been in an accident," she explained. My pre-CIA, naive brain started to engage at that point, and I asked if Estella might be studying at the university. With an odd look, she replied, coolly, "She is not a student at Georgetown." She then glanced at her daughter and requested, "Tell this man what Estella does."

"She's my nanny," the little girl replied.

It turned out that Estella was not a wealthy Venezuelan student who drove to Georgetown University in her beautiful BMW. And—surprise— she was not suffering from a brain tumor. She was just not who she said she was. That was a spectacular fail on the test for authenticity.

I was taught all my life by a kind, loving mother to trust, to give people the benefit of the doubt, to look for the good in others, and to not pry or question someone's background. A religious upbringing further instilled that in me. But the CIA, for good or for ill, undid all of that. I know that Estella would not have had a chance with post-CIA me.

The CIA taught me to look for the bad in people and to pry when necessary. Actually, to always pry. The CIA taught me to not trust anyone, especially in the beginning. I learned from others as well. President Reagan preached, "Trust but verify."[3] And a soldier friend told me, "Trust me with your life but not your money or your wife." I tend to not trust people with any of the three.

I especially don't trust people with my chocolate. I don't even trust my wife with my chocolate, for good reason. One afternoon, she actually waited until I left home to sneak into our room and eat my chocolate. (Yes, she did that.)

How to check authenticity: A young lady could visit her suitor's place of employment to confirm that he, indeed, works there in his claimed position. She can make a pretext call to an office or college department and ask to speak with him (like I did). She can innocently ask to see his work or student ID, maybe with the excuse of comparing it to her own or with feigned curiosity to see how photogenic his photo is or to check the security features (magnetic strip or chip).

If he refuses to show his ID, it could be considered a "red flag" (warning sign). He might be lying about work or about having been fired from work. A red flag might not mean she will immediately end the relationship, but it is something she should mentally record for future reference.

My high school football coach "happened" to go by the grocery store where I worked and asked my employer about me, prior to my senior year in high school. How much more important is it to know about a boyfriend and potential husband than a football player?

It is very important to know if a young man is who he says he is. Make sure he is authentic.

2. Vet him for reliability. Does he show up on time? Does he protect you? Does he follow through with what he says he will do? Does he defend you and your reputation in social situations? Does he attend his classes? Is he reliable and punctual at work?

My daughter tore the MCL in her knee during a basketball game her sophomore year. Three of her classmates decided to do a puppet show during a class Christmas program, a few days after her injury. They chose, foolishly, to base the skit on her injury: puppets reenacted her injury, falling down on the ground, screaming in pain, crying out, "My season is over!" She was disappointed in the ringleaders, of course, but she was heartbroken that some of the boys she considered friends went along with the bullying. Their results of the test for reliability? Fail.

How to check reliability: Ask him to meet at a certain time and place, maybe the school track for a run. See if he places his buddies ahead of you on his priority list. Is he there when you need him? Does he defend you when others are gossiping? What would happen if you ask a friend (who is also your "source") to say something critical about you in your group of friends, when you are absent? Does he laugh and join in the criticism? Does he wait to see how others react, wanting to see what others think before he takes a position? Or does he immediately disagree with the criticism and stand up for you?

3. Vet him for honesty. I hate liars, almost as much as I hate young men who want to date my daughter. And I especially hate young men who are liars, who also want to date my daughter.

"From the mouth of a liar, even the truth is suspect."⁴

The first quality of the Boy Scout Law is being *trustworthy,* which means honesty or integrity. But how can a young woman test a young man for truthfulness? She can listen, or rather, actively listen. Active listening means paying close attention, ignoring distractions, providing feedback, and retaining and remembering—really listening.

Susan Adams of Forbes provided an excellent review in August 2012 of a book by three former CIA officers called *Spy the Lie.*⁵ She summed up their major points as follows:

- A liar will give off subtle "whiffs," or clues, which can be detected by someone who is alert. For instance, CIA officers know that it is more difficult to remember a lie than the truth, so a liar's story will usually change over time.
- A liar will often repeat back a question when asked, trying to stall and formulate a lie: "Where was I last night?" "Who was I with last night?"
- A liar will sometimes shift into "attack mode," criticizing the young lady for not believing him: "Why are you asking? Don't you trust me?"

- A liar might use flattery, especially if he feels trapped and is looking to make an ally or establish an alibi.
- A liar will sometimes tell "little white lies" to minimize the damage or blame. But there are no little white lies. Even Mark Hacking, the murderer, admitted in a statement, "There is no such thing as a harmless lie no matter how small it is."[6]

Women are often more observant than men and are better at interpreting subtle clues. They have instincts or intuitions that can help her catch that whiff of a lie. And women can have a whole conversation with their eyes alone.

So watch his eyes. Does he look away when he tells you something suspicious? Does he flash a fake smile? Watch his body language. Does he shift his weight nervously? Be observant and trust your instincts.

Adams continued,

1. Look for deceptive behaviors and responses within the first five seconds of asking a question.
2. Someone telling the truth will say immediately and plainly that they did not commit the crime.
3. Liars often respond to questions with truthful statements that cast them in a favorable light.
4. Nonverbal cues to lying include hiding the mouth or eyes, throat clearing or swallowing, grooming gestures like adjusting shirt cuffs, shifting weight back and forth, and sweating.

How to check honesty: A young woman can tell a boy something that she knows is not completely accurate (disinformation), such as she heard he got an A on his chemistry test or that he was valedictorian of his high school. See if he goes along with an inaccurate statement or chooses to correct it. Ask him about something he had claimed previously, to see if the story matches. If he has lied about something, then pin him down. Rather than ask him, "Did you lie to me?" ask, "Why did you lie to me?" Or ask him to confirm something that you already know is true. (This works on my children!) If you already know that he cheated on you with a roommate, ask him, "Would you ever date Heather?" You might find out that he is a cheat and a liar.

4. Vet him for hostile control. In the CIA, an intelligence officer needs to know if the source is loyal and would turn down a pitch from another service; is he able to resist offers of money? Is the source indeed working with the CIA or merely available to the highest bidder? Sometimes an officer will test a source by having someone else try and recruit him under a "false flag" pitch (posing as an intelligence officer from another country). Sometimes the source passes the test, and sometimes he fails. The result of a test is often very revealing.

Find out if your boyfriend is a player. The more you date him, the more loyal he should become to you and the less he should be susceptible to "hostile control," or in civilian terms, under the control of his uncontrollable passions.

Here are some ideas for how to check loyalty: See how he acts around other women at a party, school, or work. Is he friendly or flirtatious? Does he show signs of being a player? If so, a young lady can try a false flag pitch to her boyfriend. What if she has an especially beautiful cousin who is visiting from out of town, for example? She might ask her cousin to visit her boyfriend's workplace and ask him for assistance. The cousin could possibly mention that she will be in town for a week, that she has no friends, and maybe bat her beautiful, long eyelashes at him.

Wouldn't it be interesting, even valuable, for a young woman to know if her boyfriend is susceptible to hostile control—and is disloyal, or a cheater—before she spends months or years attending proms, games, and parties with a jerk who would pursue her cousin, or any girl, if given half the chance?

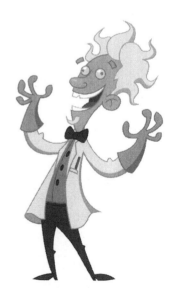

To vet someone is to look at him critically, ignoring the smile, the blue eyes, the prom tux, and the bulging biceps. She needs to examine him psychologically, emotionally, and rationally. She must find out who the person really is behind the facade, good and bad, warts and all. However handsome a young man appears in his prom tuxedo, swimsuit, football uniform, or Marine uniform, a lady must see him for who he really is, on the inside.

And if his worst is not so bad, then his not-so-bad could be good, and his good will be great. Did you follow that?

So dissect him and examine him like a scientist. Girls, be mad scientists.

Vet him for . . .

1. Authenticity. *Is he really who he says he is?*
2. Reliability. *Can you count on him?*
3. Honesty. *Does he always tell the truth?*
4. Hostile control. *Is he loyal to you, or is he constantly looking for other women?*

NOTES

1. *Avatar*, directed by James Cameron (2009, Los Angeles, CA: 20th Century Fox, 2010), DVD.

2. Antoine de St. Exupéry, *Le Petit Prince* (New York: Harcourt, 2001).

3. Old Russian proverb, adopted by Ronald Reagan during the late 1980s.

4. Unknown.

5. Susan Adams, "How to Tell When Someone Is Lying," August 13, 2012, http://www.forbes.com/sites/susanadams/2012/08/13/how-to-tell-when-someone-is-lying/.

6. *Deseret News*, Hacking Family Statement (read by Douglas Hacking, father of Mark Hacking at a press conference), June 7 2005, http://www.deseretnews.com/article/600139562/Hacking-family-statement.html?pg=all.

7
Eliciting

While I was growing up in the Salt Lake Valley, a beautiful young lady in my neighborhood married the star-football player on the Kearns High School football team. They were a charmed couple: she was classy, sweet, pretty, and intelligent, and he was handsome, athletic, and the captain of the team. It was a fairy-tale wedding of the beautiful princess to the handsome prince.

Except it was not, because he was not. During one night of their honeymoon, he crept out of their hotel room to meet his friends in a casino, get drunk, and party with ladies they had met. When she found him the next morning, hungover, she realized her mistake, but it was too late. She returned home and had the marriage annulled. It was a total disaster, not only for her, but also for her parents, his parents, and all involved.

Could knowing more about him, his personality, interests, friends, habits, and especially his character, have helped her avoid the disaster and save her a lot of misery? I think so. She could have and should have done some eliciting.

Elicitation is another art. It is an important part of spying and vetting. To elicit means to coax information from someone without his being aware of it. Elicitation might be the most important spy skill, or tool, a woman can have to learn about a young man's intentions: to read him and to find out who he really is. Elicitation skills can even help her see into the future and predict who he might become—like a real crystal ball. Real spy stuff!

Actually, many professions other than spies use elicitation:

- A lawyer uses an elicitation ploy called *assumption* during a trial, telling the defendant, "You must have been very angry when you hit him."
- A used car salesman uses a ploy called *mild provocation* when he suggests that a customer consider a lower priced model that is more "in his price range," thus offending the customer's pride and hoping to provoke a reaction. The wished-for reaction is that the customer will reveal how much he wants to spend, which might mean buying a more expensive car. The salesman is eliciting and manipulating.
- A manager might ask an applicant what he would do if he were in charge of the company. He is using the elicitation ploy called *king-for-a-day*, hoping to find out how the applicant thinks: is he a problem-solver, is he ambitious, or will he be satisfied as a fry cook. The manager is then in a better position to make a decision on whether to hire the individual or not.

As a covert operations officer, I used elicitation to find out what people wanted to tell me but were a little afraid. I sometimes learned what people did not want to tell me. I found out a lot of secret information about a lot of secret people. (No, I cannot tell you the secrets, even if you use elicitation.)

An operations officer uses elicitation a lot. He might mention to a diplomatic contact that he "heard someone say" (a ploy called *attribution*) that Government X intends to send military advisors to Country Y to eventually invade Country Z. He is hoping that the contact will confirm the report and then add more details: when, how many advisors, troops and equipment, who in the government made the decision.

A young lady who shares with a boy that she loves Taylor Swift songs is using elicitation (a ploy called *give-to-get*), hoping that the boy will admit to the same taste in music. She is looking to draw him out by sharing what she enjoys, telling him something about herself in hopes that he will do the same.

Why does a young lady have to elicit information from a young man, anyway, when she could just ask him directly? Because men, especially those with bad intentions, probably won't divulge a negative personality trait, at least not voluntarily. Asking, "Are you a stalker?" just won't work on a bad man. And a young man is also not about to come out and tell a young lady that he is addicted to pornography, is an alcoholic, or that he is working on a "100" list. He might not even voluntarily admit that he enjoys music by Taylor Swift. (Yes, I admit it.)

Eliciting, therefore, is a way to camouflage a young woman's questions as off-the-cuff observations, assumptions, or comments that are much more disarming. Elicitation allows her to then learn a lot more from his unguarded and more likely honest responses. The fun part: she can be a secret agent woman and steal his secrets, which is what covert operations officers do!

Even nice men will keep secrets. That boy at the prom with his new prom suit, haircut and aftershave is in disguise (more about this later) and is hiding secrets. In a sense, he has them all packaged up tightly with TOP SECRET stamped all over the box. So a young woman needs to unwrap the box—his personality—and make sure it contains qualities such as integrity, character, and good intentions.

To do that, she needs to learn, practice, and employ elicitation techniques. Here are ten elicitation techniques, or ploys, (some that a woman already uses without even being aware). Learn them, practice them, live them:

1. Assumption. Rather than ask a man if he plays sports, a girl can make a comment based on an observation, such as his appearance or based on something he might have said.

- If he is tall: "You look like a basketball player."
- He has big feet: "You must be a good swimmer."
- He is wearing camouflage clothes in the fall: "You look like you're going deer hunting."
- He mentions that he is from Wyoming: "I bet you're a cowboy."
- He says he has eight brothers and sisters: "I'm guessing that you are a Mormon!"
- He is handsome: "You strike me as the type of guy to have had a lot of girlfriends."
- He is wearing a new watch: "You must have received a promotion at work."
- He has a black eye: "Wow, who won the fight?"

A young man can answer the assumptions in a variety of ways, with a variety of expressions on his face: surprise, feigned humility, real humility, cockiness, or embarrassment. Assumptions are like little traps placed in front of a young man to stroll along and verbally step in. Yeah, verbal traps. I like that.

2. Give-to-get. This technique is something that we all do, even at the outset of a relationship—"Hi, my name is Dan, and I'm from Durango." We introduce ourselves with the expectation that our interlocutor will provide corresponding information, such as his name or origin. It is normal to volunteer where we are from or what school we go to. Give-to-get is also disarming because it offers an invitation to the other person. It opens the door to more conversation.

Young lady: "I love parties! I was at a party the other day that was so fun."

Young man: "Me too! I was at a party last weekend and it was out-of-control crazy. We all got so wasted, and then some neighbor called the cops, so we all had to run!"

Young lady: "Oh, I meant like my nieces' and nephews' birthday parties and Christmas parties—that sort of thing."

Later, young lady: "I enjoy fast cars! They are so exciting!"

Young man: "I was driving my dad's Corvette down the canyon the other night, going at least eighty miles per hour, with Brittany, and we were barely staying on the road. We almost went off a cliff! It was so fun!"

Young lady: "Well, I was talking about watching Nascar. Remind me to never accept a ride from you."

Give-to-get is almost as effective as Spock's mind-meld—the telepathic specialty of Spock from Star Trek—the link between his fingers and the target's brain. A young lady can effectively link to a boy's mind with simple comments about herself: her favorite movies, her interests, her aspirations, or even what she did over the weekend. Often an innocent statement can cause a young man to "spill the beans" and reveal more about himself than he intended. Or he might simply agree that he loves birthday parties . . . and Taylor Swift.

3. Attribution. Attribution is merely mentioning something as simple as "I heard that you were drinking and driving last night," or "I heard that you were a player in college." This is much harder for a Gweebi to deny or evade than if you asked him directly if he was arrested for DUI or how many girlfriends he's had. Through the use of attribution, his mind might race—*Who told her? Did she hear it from one of my friends, or* *thirdhand? How sure is she that I was arrested?* Attributing the information to an anonymous source will throw him off guard, and he could very well look at the situation as a *fait accompli* (that she already knows what happened), and he might as well confess. The odds are much higher that he will admit it when she tells him that she heard the news.

4. King-for-a-day. This ploy puts the man in a hypothetical position—a position of power—and will reveal what he would do if something were true. Asking the young man what he would do in a certain situation opens a window to his personality. It liberates him to think, dream, or speculate on what he would do in a given situation.

Young lady: "What would you do if you were Superman?"

Young man: "Well, it would be great to have X-ray vision right now!" (accompanied by creepy chuckling).

Or,

Young lady: "If you were the president of the United States, what would you do to help resolve the conflicts in the Middle East?"

Young man: "Easy, I'd drop a few nukes, kill 'em all. That's the only way to deal with those people. Want to go get a frozen yogurt?"

Young lady: "Wow. My oh my, look at the time. It is getting late, and I have a final exam in the morning. It has been fun. Buh-bye."

Or,

Young lady: "If I were in charge of the US Congress I would pass a law to raise the minimum wage." (She combines king-for-a-day and give-to-get. She has skills!)

Young Man: "Well, I would like everyone to have a living wage, but I wonder whether small businesses would survive with extra labor costs."

You just found out that he is compassionate and has some understanding of business.

5. Fragmentary. We use this ploy in hopes that a young man will complete the picture, or "fill in the blanks." She might already have the whole story about what he did last night but she wants to find out if he is truthful—if he will "tell the truth, the whole truth, and nothing but the truth." Giving a part of the story also lets him know that you are already aware of at least some of the details; he might then feel that he can't lie his way out. He might also feel compelled to provide his version or defend himself.

Young lady: "You've made out with three girls in the past few weeks. What's with that?"

Young man: "What's with what? Who says I only kissed three girls?!" (Creepy chuckle again.) "You've got to be kidding me! It was a lot more than three, and it was a lot more than kissing!"

A Gweebi, especially an arrogant one, might not be able to resist "advertising." He could either want to receive credit for his exploits and the accompanying attention he feels he deserves, or he might lie.

6. You-me-same-same. This ploy is simple—the young lady merely brings up a commonality that she might have with the young man. Commonalities, or personal connections, are great to recognize and mention when making friends and when "peeling an onion." We're all like onions, in that we peel away our own facades, insecurities, or shyness, usually layer by layer, and reveal ourselves gradually to another person. We also peel others, which can be helpful and sometimes lifesaving.

Identifying common interests, hobbies, backgrounds, or even birthplaces also deepens friendship and access. You should then use this access to get to know him better.

Woman: "Hey, I also attended Florida State University! Did you ever take Professor Smith for organic chemistry?"

Gweebi: "No way. Chemistry is way too hard. I mostly took dance, hair styling, and some singing classes. I ended up majoring in Elvis studies. Dude, it was sweet. I am now a certified Elvis impersonator!"

Or,

Woman: "I noticed you are wearing a San Diego Charger's cap. I lived there for a while."

Nice young man: "Oh yeah? I did too. I served in the Marine Corps at Camp Pendleton. I loved the weather in that area."

7. Disinformation. This technique is similar to the fragmentary ploy, except it's using false information instead of snippets of a story. Throwing out disinformation can compel a person to correct the record and reveal the truth in the process. For example, if you've heard that a boy you might date is rumored to be rough with girls, then you might say the following:

Young lady: "I heard some people at school saying (using some attribution) that you hit your last girlfriend."

Young Gweebi: "No way, she is lying. I didn't hit her. I just pushed her and she tripped over the curb. Anyway, she deserved it because she ticked me off."

8. Mild provocation. This is a favorite ploy of mine. Mildly (and I emphasize *mildly*) provoking, or "poking," someone often spurs an honest, unguarded response. Poking a tiger will provoke an angry, even violent reaction, while poking a sheep will not. Poking reveals who they really are under all that fur; a woman can find out if her friend is a tiger, a sheep, or something in between.

If you've poked a Gweebi, it could be revealing. He could become offended (if he is thin-skinned), overreact and become angry (if he has a bad temper), or laugh it off (if he is good-natured). Mild provocation can reveal a great deal about his nature and whether a girl should want to be with him or not in the future.

Mild provocation is not the same thing as being offensive. A young woman should not be rude or belittle someone. She merely wants to catch the person a little off-guard or off-balance. People make mistakes when they are a little off-balance and will unwittingly reveal secrets.

Young lady, commenting with a smile: "Your car is so old we might not make it to the theater! We'll probably break down!"

Angry young Gweebi: "Oh really? At least I have a car! You don't even have one. Anyway, my dad is going to buy me a BMW next year when I go to college, and I'll have the sweetest wheels on campus. What will you be driving?"

Or,

Woman: "You don't look so good, kind of like you didn't get much sleep last night. And what's with the hair sticking up?"

Humble man: "Yes, I was up late studying for a big physics test I took this morning. I am so beat. And I am thinking of starting a new, trendy hairstyle!"

Some of his secrets might include arrogance or humility. So poke him about his unpolished shoes, his messy hair, his wrong answer in science class, or his missed foul shot at the end of his basketball game. (Maybe wait a while if it was a big game!) Poke him like you might jab a stick in a raspberry bush to flush out any birds. Poke him and catch what secrets come flying out of his mouth.

9. Flattery. Flattery is another elicitation ploy, but it is located on the other end of the "elicitation spectrum" from mild provocation. Flattery will uncover arrogance. It is like putting a spark to a flammable ego. Flattery to a humble man will cause more blushing than anything else. Flattery to an arrogant one will just light him up!

Giving a man a compliment feeds the male ego, which is a hungry animal indeed. The male ego enjoys being fed. The arrogant male's ego demands to be fed. While compliments to a nice young man might be more embarrassing that anything, flattery to an arrogant man is more like a drug that he cannot resist.

Young lady: "Wow, what big arms you have! You must be a football player!" (Flattery, with assumption.)

Young Gweebi (wearing a shirt a few sizes too small): "Yep, I'm captain, and quarterback, and the highest scorer on our team. I was All-state for the last three years. I've had about nineteen offers from D-1 colleges around the country. I don't know which one I'll choose; they all want me so badly . . ." (thirty minutes later, still talking) ". . . and then at our homecoming game, I scored twenty-one points all on my own and won the game for our team!"

Can you imagine thirty minutes of that? Now imagine thirty years of being married to someone like that.

10. Current events. This is a common ploy in the spy business. It's a way to spark a conversation based on what's happening in the world. Using current events is merely selecting a news headline and asking about it, such as, "Isn't it tragic what's happening in . . . (pick a country). Have you heard what's happening on the US-Mexico border? The Syrian civil war? Ebola epidemic?" Bringing up a current event can uncover a lot about a person: his political views, if he is well-read, and if he is even aware of world events. She can also learn if he is aware of human tragedies, or even cares about them.

Young woman: "I read that Joe Biden visited the Ukraine last week to discuss the conflict."

Young man who does not read the news (YMWDNRN): "Uh, who's Joe Biden? What conflict? Dude, have you seen the new zombie blaster game 5? It's so awesome!"

Being familiar with, and proficient at, elicitation can save you money on a used car, help you achieve better grades in school, and facilitate finding a job or even a better-paying position. Being good at elicitation can also mean the difference between going on a date with a great guy or a stalker. Elicitation can even save your life.

Like I said, elicitation is an art. So girls, be artists.

Elicit with the following:

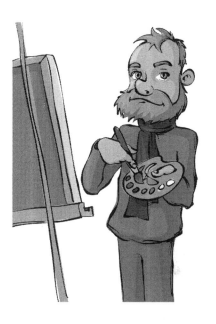

1. Assumption. *Observe, then comment.*

2. Give-to-get. *Share something about yourself.*

3. Attribution. *"I heard that . . ." or "I read that . . ."*

4. King-for-a-day. *"If you were (the boss, the president, a father), what would you do?"*

5. Fragmentary. *Give a piece of the story and let him fill in the rest.*

6. You-me-same-same. *Identify something in common.*

7. Disinformation. *Give a slightly different version of the story.*

8. Mild provocation. *Poke him.*

9. Flattery. *Compliment him.*

10. Current events. *Bring up the news.*

8

Testing

A young woman needs to test a man to effectively vet him. Most women already know how to test by nature and will check men regularly with questions like, "Do these pants make me look fat?" or, "Do you think that girl walking across the street is hot?" Of course, most men are already familiar with these common test questions, and have the answers—or lies—memorized: 1) "Heck no, you look great in anything!" and 2) "What girl?"

Men are often one step ahead of women, at least in sneakiness. I heard Jimmy Stewart tell a joke about a husband and wife having breakfast:

The wife, Margaret, asked, "If I died, would you get remarried right away?"

Her husband, John, replied, "Well, that's the darndest thing to ask. Here it's a beautiful morning and we're having a nice breakfast together, and you bring up something terrible like that. I'm not going to talk to you about that. Forget about that."

She didn't forget about it and asked later that night, "If I died, would you remarry?"

John finally relented and said, "Okay, yes, I would. Is that settled?"

Margaret continued "Well, would you sell the house?"

"No, I wouldn't," replied an increasingly perturbed John.

"Would you sell our bed?" she added.

"No, I certainly would not."

Margaret then insisted, "You certainly wouldn't let her touch my golf clubs?"

"No, no," he responded spontaneously. "She's left-handed."[1]

Why do we sometimes feel that it's too sneaky or manipulative to test someone? Testing people is actually a necessary part of life. We test people for a driver's license, for eyeglasses, to enlist in the military, to enter college, or to work at Walmart or the CIA. We are tested from preschool on. So should we feel guilty for testing a potential spouse? For testing someone who is going to be marrying my daughter? Okay, there I go again, hating.

Let's discuss some of the other criteria, or qualities, upon which a young man needs to be tested:

1. Test him for overconfidence. An arrogant young man might look at a woman through the prism of what she can do for him, even using her to make himself appear bigger, better, more attractive, or more virile. He might be thinking about how he will look to his buddies or other girls while wearing her on his arm like a Rolex watch.

A year or so ago, I passed the front desk at our local gym and spoke briefly with the lady working there. She asked me how I was doing, and I grumbled, bluntly, that I disliked coming to the gym.

"I don't like the whole environment, the mirrors, the whole atmosphere of guys walking around posing in their itsy-bitsy shirts, the vanity."

"What do you mean?" she probed.

"You must have seen the little guy that walks around here, posing, flexing, lifting weights and grunting, or heading to the tanning salon. Why does he work out?"

"Oh," she replied icily, "you mean the little guy in the body-building photo on the wall over there? You mean my husband?" (Yep, that happened to me.)

Some young men work out to be in shape, some for attention from the girls, and some for vanity. Many men follow the gym rat's motto: "Curls (exercise for biceps) for the girls." The gym might be a man's top priority in life. He might prefer to be stronger in the gym than in math or any other subject. Or he might just like to stay healthy and physically fit. A young woman needs to know which.

A divorced woman I met a few years ago confided that her husband of twenty-five years had become so obsessed with the gym—with building muscles and even taking steroids—that he had distanced himself from her. And once immersed in that world, he left her permanently for another women he met there.

A young woman who is worried about her muscle-obsessed boyfriend might want to pass along the following advice, which a high school health teacher in town shares with boys in his weight-lifting class, especially to those who spend too much time in front of the mirror, "First you fall in love with your own muscles, then with some other guy's muscles. Next thing you know, you are slathering yourself with oil and dancing around on a stage in your underwear."

Not all bodybuilders are arrogant. But a young lady needs to find out why he works out. Or why he plays a musical instrument. Or why he collects butterflies. Is he doing it to show off or for some other reason?

Does the young man project an arrogant demeanor or body language when he walks down the school hallway? Is he humble and friendly? Does he detest people who do not compliment or fawn over him? Does he have an inflated opinion of his own opinions? Does he leave room for your position on topics of discussion? Can you express your views on something that he considers himself an expert? How does he react? Is he able to see the world from your perspective, as a woman? Can he listen to your point of view, appreciate it, and appreciate you?

How to find out if he is overconfident or arrogant: Is he capable of feeling empathy? When a young lady falls in the hallway, does he fall down as well, in a laughing fit with his buddies, or does he run to help her get up? Does he feel remorse for his mistakes? Is he able to say sorry when he messes up, when he is late for a date, or has hurt your feelings? Or does he blame others?

You can try dressing-down, rather than up, on the next date or at a school party. See how he reacts when you are more a Timex than a Rolex on his arm, dressed in a frumpy outfit that you purchased at the second-hand store. Is he embarrassed to be with you, or does he still find you gorgeous and fun and has a great time during your date?

In high school, my older brother had a British sports car, a Triumph TR6. Rather than take a date in the Triumph, he would test her by arriving at her home in our beat-up Plymouth station wagon, bearing torn seats, smelling like old socks, and having popcorn in the seat cracks. He wanted to find out if she was attracted to him or the car.

Arrogant, narcissistic people feel an overpowering need to be the center of attention. And they can be thin-skinned. So go to a party and show him less attention than usual, maybe ignore him at times or show others more attention than him. Does his jealousy grow to anger? Is he borderline violent? Any hint of a violent reaction is a definite fail on this test and should end any potential relationship.

2. Test him for underconfidence. Men who lack confidence, especially to the point of having an inferiority complex, can be difficult to live with. Strangely enough, a young man lacking confidence can act overconfident.

A relative of mine, a standout in track, once dated a young man who also competed in track but wasn't as successful. He was a good athlete in his own right, but he became somewhat resentful of her times and distances, some of which surpassed his. She eventually grew tired of his boasting or excuses (sore back, sun was in my eyes, and so on), and they stopped dating.

Admittedly, dating her would be tough on any young man's ego. She eventually married another outstanding athlete who also has a healthy level of confidence. Problem solved.

> **"No one is more arrogant toward women, more aggressive or scornful, than the man who is anxious about his virility."**
>
> **—Simone de Beauvoir[2]**

How to find out if a man lacks confidence: observe how he walks around the office or campus, how he talks to peers, how he communicates with business associates, or how he interacts with others. Granted, many men are somewhat shy and lacking in confidence at a young age but will gain confidence and turn out fine as they mature. But learn to recognize young men who feel negative about their own abilities and might either resent or mistreat you. How does he react to your successes? Achievement of classmates? How does he react when you compliment others? Or his teammate? Or a competitor from another school's team: "Wow, that basketball player from the opposing team did not miss a shot!" Does he become overly jealous, angry, or bitter?

3. Test him for kindness and compassion. How does he treat little furry animals? Small children? Older adults? People with disabilities? How does he treat your friends? Waiters? People that he might consider "below" him? Raytheon CEO Bill Swanson wrote a booklet of thirty-three leadership observations called *Swanson's Unwritten Rules of Management*. Rule number thirty-two states, "A person who is nice to you but rude to the waiter, or to others, is not a nice person. (This rule never fails.)"[3]

Observe how the young man treats his mother. How does he behave around his sister? If he's different with them, if he mistreats them, don't tell yourself that lots of boys are that way with their mothers, or that it's normal for a boy to yell at his mom. Don't make excuses for his swearing at his sister by calling it sibling rivalry. Eventually, he will treat you the same way that he treats others.

How to find out if he is kind and compassionate: Tell him you are going to volunteer at the local assisted living center or daycare center, and ask if he'd like to go along. Invite him when you visit your grandma, or when you take young nephews to play at the playground. Get up from dinner at Grandma's and immediately start clearing the dishes to see if he helps out or stays put and starts talking football with your lazy brothers. Invite him to interact with people that can do nothing for him in terms of furthering his education, his résumé, or his career. And observe.

Observe how many times he checks his watch, his text messages, or the clock on the wall, all because he is anxious to leave. Observe how he reacts when a toddler suffering from a cold wipes snot on his new shirt. Is he understanding and laughs it off, or does he react angrily?

Some guys might be able to fake it during an outing with a young woman's grandma, hoping to earn "points," or a "reward" for their kindness. It might just be another down payment. So use your intuition, your spy skills, and catch him—steal his secrets! A young women with spy skills might enlist friends—her sources, unknown to the young man—who can report how he acts when she isn't around: at the church picnic, in the locker room, or when he is in the park with his buddies, all kicking a puppy or telling dirty jokes. How does he act when you are not around? It had better be the same way that he acts when he is with you, or he fails this test.

And make sure the test is a "double-blind" test. In other words, do not give extra "Brad Pitt-hottie" points to someone who's not kind or compassionate to people he feels are below him. (Refer back to rule number thirty-two). Be rational rather than rationalize. What a difference that little ending, -ize, can make in a word!

4. Test him for patience. This is a challenging quality for me, and I often fail this test. I am not particularly patient. But a girl must learn how patient her boyfriend or fiancé is at this stage in his life.

I feel that most of our emotions, qualities, or weaknesses are connected, as if in a personality "chain." If I'm right, then patience is connected to strength, endurance, determination, and success. Impatience can lead to frustration, anger, jealousy, anxiety, and even failure.

> **"It is easier to find men who will volunteer to die, than to find those who are willing to endure pain with patience."**
>
> **—Julius Caesar[4]**

There are many ways to tell if someone is patient. Walk slow. Talk slow! "Accidentally" change the channel before the end of an exciting play of the football game. Stop to tie your shoe when you are both rushing to class. Take him hiking and purposely forget the water (maybe not if you are hiking in Death Valley in the summer!), to see who he becomes when he's hot and thirsty or when an activity is not going according to plan. Does he blame you and swear in frustration? That would be a fail. Or does he just shake his head and maybe feel a little embarrassed that he forgot to bring water? Try being intentionally late for your date and make him wait. Does he tease you good-naturedly or react with impatience and anger?

Observe what he is like when he loses a state championship baseball game—is he just frustrated or furious? Does he whisper to you with a sad but courageous smile, "We'll get them next year." That would be a pass.

5. Test him for impulse control. "Tiger Mom" Amy Chua, who wrote *The Triple Package*, argues that some groups in America do better than others based on "a cultural edge" that enhances their ability to succeed. One of the three traits Chua identifies is "impulse control." She explains, "Impulse control refers to the ability to resist temptation, especially the temptation to give up in the face of hardship or quit instead of persevering at a difficult task."[5]

Is he able to resist impulses or temptations? Does he devour every doughnut at the party? Is he able to resist going to a party and decide, instead, to stay home and study for a final exam? (My niece's husband would regularly ask her if she had finished her homework before going on a date with her.) Will the young man sleep in rather than help a friend move to a new apartment? Can he resist looking at vulgar photos that someone sends him on his iPhone? Or pornography? Is he able to skip an evening of video games with his buddies in order to work at a service project?

6. Test him for frugality. Not too long ago, 89 percent of divorces were due to differences, arguments, and fights over money. Maybe the percentage is even higher now. Sonya Britt, an assistant professor of family studies and human services at Kansas State University conducted a study on 4,500 couples and found that "arguments about money is by far the top predictor of divorce. It's not children, sex, in-laws or anything else. It's money—for both men and women."[6]

A woman needs to learn if her boyfriend, or potential husband, is compatible in financial terms. She needs to know if he so tight with money that he needs to "unscrew his wallet" to buy an ice cream cone. Or is she the one who has to unscrew her purse to buy anything at a second-hand store and he the spendthrift? Whatever the mix, a young lady needs to find out the young man's thoughts on money, on saving versus spending, and on credit cards. Especially credit cards and other debt as well.

She needs to know if he will add $100,000 in student loans to the marriage—maybe with additional credit card debt on top of that. She might still marry him, but she needs to have her eyes wide open in terms of financial responsibilities, especially liabilities.

Is he willing to forgo luxury items (nice car, clothes, the latest cell-phone) until he can afford them? She might volunteer information on her own financial situation (give-to-get), inviting him to divulge information on his finances. If that doesn't work, she could point out that she was also a student (you-me-same-same) and mention that she and her parents paid for her schooling . . . hint, hint . . . sure hope that your school costs have been paid too.

If he won't open up about finances and you're getting serious or are engaged to be married, then ask him directly: How much debt are you carrying? How many credit cards do you have? How much do you have in savings? Assets? Stocks?

Ask, ask, ask. You tried eliciting, now it is time to learn the whole story before it's too late. It's more important than finding out how many children he wants, more important than finding out if his in-laws want to move in to the home next door, more important than "anything else," according to the above study.

7. Test him for respect. A friend of mine talked about a young woman that had been going on casual dates with two young men during the same period of time. One seemed to always make her the butt of jokes, teasing her relentlessly, while the other young man was more respectful.

I was warned many times by my mother to stop teasing my wife and my children. I find it annoying when I am the target of teasing, so I can only imagine how others feel.

Respect seems to be a vanishing commodity, or quality, in our society. It is getting more rare to see a young man offer to give up his seat for an elderly individual or for a young man to say "excuse me" when he walks between two people. But even though manners seem to be old-fashioned, both men and women still appreciate it. It's not old-fashioned to open a door for someone else, or say "excuse me," or put a hand over your mouth when you yawn. Respect will always be in fashion.

How to test him for respect: see how he treats his parents, his teachers, and his elders. Does he stand and offer a pregnant lady his seat on the bus? Does he listen to senior citizens or snicker when they struggle with a memory? Does he have respect for others who are different? Does he respect our military or the flag? What is he doing during the playing of the National Anthem? Take him to a city council meeting. Take him to church. Take him to a hospital. Take him to a Fourth of July parade. Is he respectful?

8. Test him for work ethic. Work is another quality that seems to be in short supply. I was so pleased that my oldest son found a job with a boss who knew how to really inspire work in his employees. The company installs geothermal heating and cooling systems for large buildings, and my son found himself working in dirt trenches, shoveling in one hundred–plus temperatures, sometimes for sixteen-plus hours a day when the company needed to finish the job before the next stage of construction. I felt sorry for my son during those hot days but also pride and gratitude that he was learning the meaning of hard work.

My son didn't always understand the meaning of work. When he was about four years old I took him to a park to play. In between swings and slides he came over to me and said, "Papa, you know how you go to the office for your job?" I replied in the affirmative, and he responded, with a nod toward the playground, "Well, this is my job."

A young lady needs to find out if her future spouse knows the difference between playing and working. And while playground tester, computer gamer, or chocolate taster would all be great jobs, there just aren't that many positions available. If there were more chocolate taster positions available, then I know someone who would be living in Belgium and gaining a lot of weight. Me.

He needs to know how to work and be willing and able to work hard to support his family and future children. The expression "deadbeat" dad has become all too common a term. Although it usually refers to divorced fathers, there are plenty of married fathers who are failing to take care of their families.

How to test him for work ethic: a young lady can see how the young man spends his summers. Is he usually at the beach, bumming most of his days away, or does he work a job or two? If he doesn't, invite him to go help a neighbor do yard work or help find him a job.

Does he have chores at home? A friend who owns a local Dairy Queen told our group of disabled job seekers that she typically asks an applicant if he has chores at home. If he admits to having none, then he most likely will not get the job. Another employer asks his applicants about their extracurricular activities at school and loves to hear that an applicant is a cross-country runner; it indicates he's disciplined enough to wake up early in the morning during the summer months. It shows self-discipline and mental and physical toughness.

9. Test him for violent tendencies. Not every young man who spends a lot of his time playing violent video games is violent by nature. These young men who are addicted to watching violence may not become murderers or rapists. Most of them won't. We hope. But as they spend lots and lots of time fantasizing about shooting people in increasingly realistic, violent video games, they might not be particularly upset at the sight of violence. They've seen it so many times, thousands of murders, and murdered thousands, maybe millions, of virtual people. Ain't no big thing.

By the way, if images don't have any effect on people at all, then companies must be wasting a lot of money on advertising hamburgers and beer during football games. Images affect us all, to some degree or another.

A young lady needs to find out if a young man has a bad temper or can become violent if things do not go his way. And she should hope to find out if he has violent tendencies before he tries the violence on her. See how he reacts when he's angry. Find his boiling point. I'm not suggesting that you intentionally provoke him to anger, but watch him carefully during stressful, frustrating situations. Does he become aggressive while driving in traffic? Playing sports? When he burns his toast? When he hits his thumb with a hammer? Be observant.

10. Test him for compatibility. Do you share interests, habits, commonalities, or goals with him? Do you share core values? Does he enjoy watching Shakespeare or professional wrestling? MMA or ballet? Neither my wife nor I enjoy the opera. We once walked out of an opera in a wonderful concert hall in Paris, France, during intermission. (Yes, we did that.) Unfortunately, or fortunately, we're both compatible concerning our taste in opera. And our taste in chocolate.

A couple does not have to share every interest. Variety is the spice of life, after all, and spouses can bring a variety of skills, interests, or hobbies to a marriage, which will enrich the other and their life together; my wife enjoys cooking and I bake bread. But a couple should share important values such as views on religion or raising children or whether to have children at all. Too often a couple will fall in love (or lust) over shared interests in music, Indian food, or opera, but later find out that they do not share views on the important stuff.

Compatibility includes a good sense of humor! Does she like to laugh, while he's about as funny as a heart attack? Seriously, I would find it dreadful to date, let alone marry, someone who doesn't have a sense of humor. Humor allows us to laugh when we trip and fall down the church steps, vomit on a friend's carpet, or chop our fingers off in the lawn mower. (Well, maybe not that last one.) We'll all have flat tires in a thunderstorm, get fired by our fat boss at the health food store, break bones crashing on our bicycle, and pass gas in bed. A sense of humor insulates and inoculates a relationship from heartache and from life when it happens—and it does, and it will.

So test him with some jokes, like, "How do we know that Adam was a Mormon? (Because only a Mormon could stand next to a naked lady and be tempted by a piece of fruit!) What did the pirate say when he turned eighty? (Aye matey! Get it? I'm eighty!)" If he doesn't laugh at those jokes, then he has no sense of humor. Or he doesn't get the joke, which means that you need to test him on intelligence.

Compatibility in a couple is crucial. If she's bubbly and he only enjoys popping her bubbles, there will be problems in any future relationship. Does she enjoy classical music, while he enjoys belching "The Star-Spangled Banner"? Does she like to dance and he has two left-feet? An aunt of mine complained that she had not danced with her husband since they were married—for fifty, long years.

No young man can pass all of these tests, but the guy you should date, or end up marrying, should do well on balance. So begin to test him as soon as possible because it takes time, and a young lady needs to conduct lots of tests.

Girls, test him. Test him like an ornery, disgruntled staffer at the Department of Motor Vehicles testing a teenager!

Test him for the following:

1. Overconfidence
2. Underconfidence
3. Kindness and compassion
4. Patience
5. Impulse control
6. Frugality
7. Respect
8. Work ethic
9. Violent tendencies
10. Compatibility

NOTES

1.   Jimmy Stewart, "Funniest Joke I ever Heard 1984," YouTube, www.youtube.com/watch?v=3IiICcSH8iY.

2.   Simone de Beauvoir, "Introduction: Woman as Other," *The Second Sex* (New York: Vintage, 2011).

3.   William H Swanson, *Swanson's Unwritten Rules of Management* (Waltham: Raytheon, 2005).

4.   Jon R. Stone, *The Routledge Dictionary of Latin Quotations* (New York: Routledge, 2004), 307.

5.   Amy Chua, *The Triple Package* (London: Penguin Books, reissued 2015).

6.   Kansas State University "Researcher Finds Correlation Between Financial Arguments, Decreased Relationship Satisfaction," last modified July 12, 2013, http://www.k-state.edu/media/newsreleases/jul13/predictingdivorce71113.html.

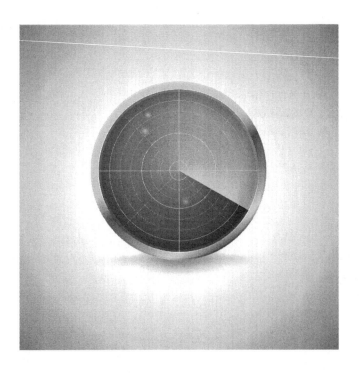

9

Demeanor

An aircraft that never appears on an enemy's radar screen has a much better chance of survival. This aircraft that flies by stealth, under the radar, will most likely never even have a missile fired at it, let alone be forced to make evasive maneuvers to avoid being shot down.

The same thing goes for a covert operations officer—avoiding enemy radar is a top priority.

Espionage operations need to be carried out undetected, quietly, often under the nose of a host country. It's a sneaky, stealthy business. Many people believe that the day-to-day work of a covert operations officer involves James Bond types driving fasts cars, flirting with fast women, shooting bad guys, swimming underwater to enter a castle controlled by an evil megalomaniac, jumping out of planes without a parachute, playing poker with evil geniuses while being poisoned, and emerging from cryogenic freezing to combat blonde "fem-bots" firing automatic weapons from a bra. Wait, that was Austin Powers.

But you get the picture. That is the Hollywood version. In real life, intelligence officers want to avoid all the fracas, shooting, bombs, and brassiere blasters. In real life, spies stay off the radar and therefore avoid scrutiny, detection, and even becoming a target in the first place.

For spies and young ladies, demeanor plays a big part in staying off the radar. And dah-meaner, dah-better!

Seriously, demeanor, or a person's conduct, can mean the difference between a predator targeting a young woman because he considers her an easy target—a soft target—or a predator deciding that she is a hard target and someone not worth the trouble of pursuing. Just as a woman can assess a man according to his demeanor, so can a sexual predator or stalker judge a young lady based upon hers. He can ascertain a lot simply watching her walk past him on the street. Is she . . .

- confident or shy?
- brave or afraid?
- purposeful or unsure where she is going, even lost?
- strong or weak?
- happy or upset?
- vulnerable or not vulnerable?

A predator can look at a woman and assess her based on her clothes, body language, posture, and even the pace of her walking. It might be a snap judgment, but predators can do it quickly, much as a lioness scanning a herd of zebras. A lioness can pick out the injured, the weak, the sick, the tired, the young, and zero in on a vulnerable zebra almost instantly. Human predators can do the same thing, only they're no longer the little boys in the neighborhood, watching her from the bushes across the street; they're now lions . . . with teeth.

A young lady walking home across campus with her shoulders back, head erect, eyes alert, paying attention to her surroundings (not staring at her cellphone), and moving at a brisk pace is much less likely to attract targeting than a lady who is shuffling along, eyes fixed on the sidewalk or her cellphone, possibly struggling to carry a backpack full of books, or projecting an image of being oblivious to her surroundings.

An oblivious, scared-looking, lost woman while walking through the wrong neighborhood will be more vulnerable to bad men: stalkers, rapists, and thugs. It's the law of the jungle. I'm not saying that she's inviting an assault, or "got what she deserved," as some idiots would suggest. I would never blame the victim for an assault or rape but only for allowing herself to appear distracted, weak, or distraught, and therefore become more vulnerable.

Walk with confidence. Now a young lady might say to herself, "I'm not confident, so I can't walk that way or appear confident." Yes, you can! Even if you don't feel confident, you can fake it! If you need to, practice walking at home in front of the mirror or in front of your family or friends. Throw your shoulders back, hold your head erect, and walk! Confidence is like everything else in life that we are trying to learn. We all practice and just fake it in the beginning. We fake piano, football, and algebra while we're learning. Tell yourself to walk across campus, down a street, or across the stage, and then fake it.

Some say, "fake it 'til you make it." I do it all the time. I did it in the CIA. I did it as a substitute teacher, as a job coach for disabled kids, as a member of the ski patrol, and even as a carpenter. And I still have all my fingers! Everyone does this at one time or another. I'm actually faking being a writer right now, as I type this. Maybe I will be a confident writer someday.

To gain confidence, a young lady can tell herself that she is a precious young woman. She can choose to believe that. She can choose confidence, just like she chooses to have hope and happiness. If she needs to, she can tell herself, "I'm a good friend to others. I'm a good artist. I'm a fine musician." She can also listen to those who support her rather than those who tear her down. The people who criticize are no more correct or factual than friends and family who build you up. Who is right? You can choose who is right!

So try on a little confidence and wear it around. And then take that little confidence outfit and walk downtown (during the day), even if you're not quite sure. Walk into that Dairy Queen like you own the place. And order yourself a hamburger—hold the pickles and any self-doubt—with a side order of courage. And then walk to your car like you own it, because you do! And then do it again the next day. And the next.

That's how people become self-assured: little by little, fake by fake. Until you convince yourself that you are self-assured, as much as any of the other nervous humans walking around on this planet.

Walk with a purpose. Even if you're lost, walk as if you know where you're going. I can't imagine how many tourists in far-off countries have been robbed, beaten, kidnapped, or raped because they walked out of an airport or subway station looking like lost puppies. Tourists often shuffle around cities with their heads down, eyes fixed on a map, or staring up at the big map on the subway wall, heads turning this way and that, all obvious foreigners with worried looks on their foreign faces. Their demeanor is practically screaming to pickpockets and any number of other predators looking for easy prey.

Female students who walk across campus with a lost demeanor can attract the unwanted attention of a would-be stalker. He might spot her after a few steps down the sidewalk if she acts lost. He might even ask her if she needs assistance.

So if a young lady is walking in an environment in which she's not familiar or comfortable, she can walk to a certain location—the campus library, for instance—and away from where a would-be assailant wants her, which is at a lonely bus stop or in a tree-covered walkway. She can walk to the bookstore, a restaurant, or a government building. Then she can stand or sit with her back against the wall, her purse under her arm, and look at her map.

Last, do not become distracted. Most magic tricks depend on distraction in order to be successful. A magician uses one hand to distract while the other pulls an item out of his pocket. It is difficult to watch both. Do not let yourself be distracted when walking or driving in an area you're not familiar with.

Do not be distracted by texting or talking on a cell phone. You won't be aware of your surroundings (ditches, open manholes, stop signs, cracks in the sidewalk) or aware of people around you. You won't be aware of people who might be targeting you. In May 2015, a viral video showed a stalker following a thirteen-year-old girl to the front porch of her home before she noticed him and then fought him off inside her door. What the news stories didn't mention, however, is that the young girl was completely engrossed in her cell phone, texting as she walked.

The same advice goes for using cell phones in all public areas: if you receive a text or phone call while walking in an area where you're not comfortable, walk inside a restaurant, or library, or store, put your back to a wall away from the door, and then read your text, send your reply, or call. If someone is watching you and sees you move like that, he will most likely tell himself, "I'm not going to mess with her."

I don't know what it's like to be a woman. But I do know that it must be wonderful to be a woman (especially Wonder Woman). So don't let a predator even think that he could take advantage of you if you come up on his radar. Project an image of confidence. Walk past him like you would defend yourself if he ever tried anything harmful. If he is someone with bad intentions, then he could leave you alone

> **"I'd much rather be a woman than a man. Women can cry, they can wear cute clothes, and they're the first to be rescued off sinking ships."[1]**
>
> **—Gilda Radner**

and watch you go on your way, just because of the demeanor you project.

A young woman's demeanor can tell all men she encounters that she is confident, purposeful, not to be trifled with, not vulnerable, and not a target. Even a good man will decide that she is not to be treated lightly, and that he had better be on his best behavior.

Her demeanor will send a message well before any targeting has taken place, like a porcupine's demeanor—and quills—tell a predator don't mess with me. So be a porcupine.

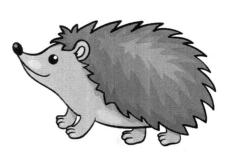

Project an image of . . .

1. Confidence
2. Purpose
3. Alertness

Do not be distracted.

NOTES

1. Dailycaller.com, "Comedians Who Died Too Young," accessed August 10, 2015, http://dailycaller.com/2014/04/15/comedians-who-died-too-young-slideshow/gildaradner-1980/.

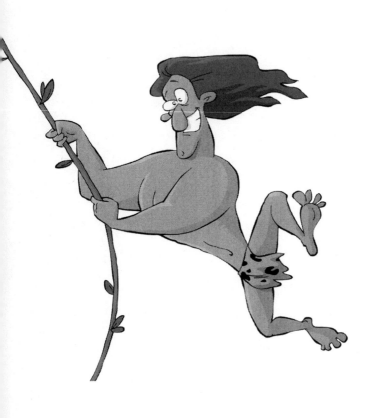

10

Tarzan and Jacqueline

"I am Tarzan of the Apes. I want you. I am yours. You are mine. We live here together always in my house. I will bring you the best of fruits, the tenderest deer, the finest meats that roam the jungle. I will hunt for you. I am the greatest of the jungle fighters. I will fight for you. I am the mightiest of the jungle fighters."[1] —Tarzan

I was always captivated with Africa—the Dark Continent, as they used to call it—since my childhood. When I was young, my family would gather in front of our black-and-white TV every Friday night, bowls of popcorn on our TV trays, ready to watch Johnny Weissmuller play Tarzan. We watched him every week as he saved Jane from lions and crocodiles, beat his chest, and screamed his jungle scream. I even learned to beat my chest and scream like him. I was Tarzan, in my mind, saving my future wife.

In March 1988, twenty-five years after I first watched Tarzan on TV, I was sitting at the side of a swimming pool at the Okapi Hotel in Kinshasa, Zaire, now called Democratic Republic of the Congo. While I might not have been wearing a loincloth made from antelope like my hero, I was in Africa as I had always dreamed.

And right across the swimming pool sat a young woman who I had also dreamed about: dark hair, dark eyes, as beautiful a woman as I had ever seen. Even more beautiful than Jane.

But while she was only a short walk away, she might as well have been on Mt. Everest. I just couldn't find the courage to stand up and walk over there. So I watched her, surveilled her, and studied her, all the while wrestling with myself, with my inner Tarzan:

"Ungawa, me Tarzan, she Jane."

"Whoa, hang on to your loincloth, buddy. You don't even know her."

"Ungawa (he said that a lot), Tarzan want. Talk woman."

"Nah, waste of time. A lady that beautiful must have a boyfriend."

"Me greatest jungle fighter. Me take Jane from boyfriend!"

The Tarzan in me finally got up and walked around to her side of the pool. My legs felt encased in cement, I was so nervous. As I approached, I noticed that two young men were playing volleyball next to her, hitting the ball directly over her, trying their best to get her attention. It was an amateur tactic.

My approach was not much better than theirs. I was an amateur at pick-up lines in English, and more so in my rudimentary French. I must have sounded a lot like Tarzan to her:

"Men bother you, I save you. You come with me?"

"Oh, no thanks, I'm fine right here," she replied.

Unprepared for her response, and unsure what to do next, I sat down beside her and tried again.

"Me man, you woman. I eat you for dinner when sun sets?"

"Well, um, no thanks. Afraid I'm busy tonight."

"I want we go hunt meat. Two dark times?"

"Really? No, I can't go tomorrow either, sorry."

"Ungawa, we eat best fruits and finest meats, in three dark times?"

Seriously, I really did have to ask her out three times, suggesting three different nights, before she finally relented. With no CIA training whatsoever, she "tested" me for several things, including courage, respect, and even determination. She also sent me a message: that she would not rush into a date with a stranger, that she was special, and that I would have to be on my best behavior. The whole conversation was more involved than described above, and more information was exchanged between the "no thank yous," but that was the gist of our conversation—I was going to have to work hard for a date with her.

Interestingly, I learned that traditional Chinese often decline a gift three times before they will accept. I like that. I think that I will start that practice, to decline a gift three times, unless it's chocolate.

I didn't know it at the time, but my future life hung by a thread during this initial examination or vetting. And I almost quit before my last attempt, but I pressed on. Maybe it was how she looked in a swimsuit. Maybe it was inspiration from my eighth grade French teacher, Mrs. Potter, who first struggled to teach me French, and later, Professor Mills in college.

But twenty years later, here I was, using French with an African beauty, and she had finally replied *"oui."* That *oui* erased all those embarrassing years battling verb conjugations and struggling to pronounce that French *r*. My teachers would have been proud!

I somehow managed to wait for the three "dark times" and drove downtown to pick her up. We ate dinner at the Western Steak restaurant, located on Boulevard de Trente Juin, in downtown Kinshasa. We had a wonderful conversation and talked about everything under the sun. Miraculously, she was able to interpret my Tarzan French. I ordered

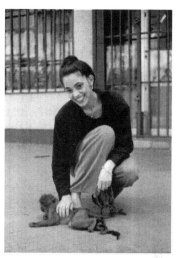

My wonderful wife, in Kinshasa, Democratic Republic of the Congo.

baked python, of course, just as Tarzan would have done. (Yes, I really did.)

Before we parted that night, I wanted to do what most men do—I tried to kiss her. Always the optimist, I actually figured that her first *oui* meant more *oui*'s to come. I was wrong. As I moved in, she deftly turned her head at the last second, blocking me with her cheek. It was a classy but frustrating move.

She made me wait. She was already training me to be a gentleman. And I made sure to act the gentleman and be careful after that.

I remember being careful one evening in Hawaii a few years earlier, while attending a university there. I visited a Samoan home to take a young lady, Mele, on a date. When I entered her living room, her cousin invited me to sit down. As I found a chair, I greeted her very large Samoan father, who was wearing a lavalava, and her mother seated next to him. There were other equally large relatives seated along the walls.

When Mele entered, she sat down next to me but did not say a word or give any indication that she was ready to leave. We sat in awkward silence for a few moments until the cousin hissed at me, whispering, "Hey brah (a Hawaiian expression that is short for "brother"), you need to ask him."

"Ask him what?" I replied, clueless.

"You got to ask if you can date his daugh-tah," he said back, chuckling.

I hadn't expected this, but I forged ahead.

"Sir," I managed to cough out, "is it okay if I take your daughter on a date?"

"Where you go?" he shot back with an angry look.

"I plan to take her to Honolulu to go—"

"TOO FAH," he boomed.

After a few seconds, his wife whispered to him in Samoan. It appeared to me that she was playing the role of referee.

"When you come home?" he asked again, rather menacingly. He looked a lot like my friend Joe looks at boys who want to date his daughters, like he hated me.

I thought quickly and answered, "We should be back by midnight because—"

"TOO LATE" he yelled.

Again, his wife spoke to him, appearing to calm him down. After a few more minutes, he eventually agreed with a nod of his head, but with a frown still frozen on his face.

I had Mele home at 11:30. There was no sitting and kissing on my motorcycle in their driveway. There was no monkey business. Nothing. Nothing but fear, respect, and being careful.

The day after my careful date with Jacqueline, I bought her flowers from one of the road-side vendors, to say *merci*, but mainly just as an excuse to see her again. And also because I had to ask her out three times, and she had turned her cheek when I tried to kiss her, and now I had to prove to her that I was indeed a gentleman.

It's interesting how that works. In one day, she had already begun training me to be on my best behavior. Ladies can do that for a young man. And she told me later that she had appreciated the flowers.

The night before I left the Congo, Jacqueline and her mother prepared a fine African meal as a farewell gesture and to celebrate my thirtieth birthday, which was the next day. The food was incredible: several dishes of peanut chicken (still one of my favorites), rice, pondu, and fufu. If it was the flowers that worked their charm on Jacqueline, it was partly the food that worked on me. She was an incredible cook.

As I was driving with Jacqueline and her mother on the day of my departure, I jokingly told her mother, "I think that I might take your daughter with me to America."

"No, no, no," she quietly replied. Another no; like mother, like daughter.

The next day, the day of my birthday, after having flown from Kinshasa to another African country, I found myself in a room of a hotel, on the outskirts of the capital. My colleagues and I were resting up, preparing for the coming week. I had all weekend to rest and to agonize about who I had just left behind in Kinshasa.

As I stared at the hotel room ceiling, pining, I switched on the hotel TV and noticed a movie playing on the hotel channel—*Made in Heaven*. The plot involves a young man named Elmo (Timothy Hutton) who dies and goes to heaven, where he falls in love with a lady named Annie (Kelly McGillis). Unfortunately, Annie has not yet had a turn to come to earth and soon leaves, to be born and start her life. Elmo pleads with God for a chance to go back to earth again, to find her. God finally relents and gives Elmo, after some negotiating, thirty years to find her. After a bunch of near misses, Elmo finds Annie on his thirtieth birthday.

I'm not superstitious, but seeing that movie on my thirtieth birthday, the day after leaving Jacqueline, I wondered if someone was trying to tell me something.

After another month, I was back in the United States and trying to continue a relationship with another young lady. (Yes, I did that.) I was actually dating a young lady when I met Jacqueline. It took a week or so after my return before my then-girlfriend asked me what was wrong and why I was acting strange. I admitted that I had met someone during my trip to Africa. And that was that.

The next nine months were consumed by more trips, letters, phone calls, and trying to forget Jacqueline. Tarzan wanted her, but the rest of me argued that she was from a different country, continent, hemisphere, culture, religion, and racial make-up—different, different, different. It would never work. Some relatives and friends joined in the chorus—telling me to wake up, that I had jungle fever, that we were not compatible. Colleagues at work wondered why I was falling for a foreigner and warned that I was risking my career.

But at the end of those nine months, Jacqueline came to visit me in America. And it was as if we had never been apart. We fell in love, again. We traveled to Utah to introduce her to my family. Although she could not really communicate with my parents and siblings, she fell in love with them, and they with her.

She later told me that she first knew she should marry me when she met my family. Remember that, young men (if you're still reading this,

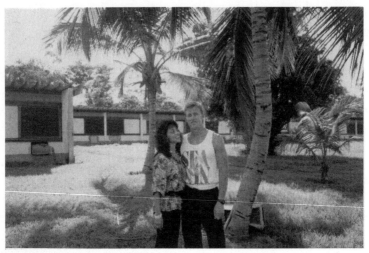

The first week Jacqueline and I met.

even after all the warnings): it might be her cooking for you, but it's flowers and family if you want to reach a woman's heart.

She returned to Africa much too soon. More long months of letters and phone calls followed. But, as luck would have it, I was able to return to Kinshasa in June 1989, after six months. Dates at more restaurants, more baked python. Dancing.

And then came our first fight. I don't really remember what it was about, but I remember driving the next morning to the bank where she worked, with every intention of breaking up with her. I was ready to let her have it. I told her that the relationship wasn't working and that we probably ought to stop seeing each other. I was ready for her tears and begging to begin.

But she didn't beg. Actually, she didn't put up much of a fight at all. She was very agreeable. I remember thinking that my plan was not going at all according to plan. I decided, instantly to give her another chance and keep seeing her. (Yes, I actually thought that.)

I departed Kinshasa again. Another nine months passed. I spoke with Jacqueline's father on the phone to convince him that I had honorable intentions. She gave away most of her belongings and departed Kinshasa with her suitcases. On the way to America, she had an overnight layover in Brussels, where she visited with her sisters. I called her that night to see how her trip was progressing.

It was then that we realized that we had not spoken about or planned where she would reside in Virginia, before our wedding. I've never been much of a planner.

"Where will I stay?" she asked.

"I guess you can stay in my place, in the other bedroom with my roommates," I replied.

"What? You have roommates? And you want me to stay with them?"

"Sure, Wendy and Noleen are two friends that rent one of the rooms in my condo."

"Your roommates are girls?" she asked, icily. I think that I actually saw frost begin to form on my telephone.

I tried to reason with her. "Well, I don't think of them as women, exactly. They are friends. I've known Wendy since college—she's like my sister. I travel a lot and they look after the place while I'm gone."

All the warnings from Jacqueline's friends about Mormons and polygamy and her not knowing what she was getting into must have echoed in her ears. Her voice changed, her mood changed. There was no more joy about her trip. As a matter of fact, she was now reconsidering coming to America at all. I can't blame her. In hindsight, I could have broached that subject a little sooner.

After some tap dancing and pleading, she agreed to come. Now I had three female roommates and an angry Mormon mom. I'm not sure about my Baptist dad's reaction. Maybe it was a fist pump.

But finally, after almost two years, countless close calls, and having brought the love of my life from the other side of the world, we still couldn't get married. There was this little matter of me working for the CIA. The CIA had to approve of the marriage to a foreigner. They had to conduct a background investigation on her. And there was the lie detector, or polygraph, test.

Most people don't know how terrifying the polygraph can be. It's very uncomfortable, and purposely so. Jacqueline was scared to death. She had grown up in a country under dictator rule, and his regime enforced that rule ruthlessly.

Her polygraph examination didn't go well. She didn't like the intrusive nature of the test, and she didn't like the person administering the test. And of course, polygraphers aren't known for being warm and fuzzy friends during the examination.

During the next six months, I continued traveling overseas. She decided to go to Belgium, thinking that she could visit her sisters again while I was gone. That plan backfired when the airlines and immigration denied her entry back into the States. I flew to Belgium, before my next mission, and tried to convince the consulate officer to give her a visa. The answer was no. Another trip to Eastern Europe, back to Belgium, and with a little help, we eventually had her visa and were able to return to America.

After another trip overseas, I returned to learn that I still didn't have approval from the CIA. Unfortunately, we had scheduled a wedding date, and I unwisely intended to stick with it. I informed my boss that I was leaving for Utah in a few days to get married. The next thing I knew, I was sitting down with another supervisor.

"Listen," he warned, "the answer is no. You're going to ruin your career with the CIA if you go through with this marriage."

"Well, so be it. I can't continue like this, with her living in my condo with two other women, an angry mom wondering what I'm doing."

"Look," he replied, "don't be crazy."

"I might be. I just have to marry this girl. And the CIA will have to do what it has to do."

At that point, he said something that I have never forgotten. "You can always find another wife, but you cannot find another job like this."

After a moment of surprise, I replied, "I think that you meant to say that I can always find another job, but I will never find another wife like this."

He stuck with his opinion, and I stuck with mine. And I flew to Utah a day later. Two days before my wedding, I got a call from another supervisor (there are lots of supervisors in the government). He advised that the CIA had given me "conditional approval."

"What the heck is that?" I asked him. He replied that it was a six-month, conditional, "probationary" thing—nothing to worry about—that I should go ahead and get married, that everything would be fine.

So I did just that. Jacqueline and I were married in a little church across the street from my family home. She was late for the wedding, of course, but stunning. She's been late to almost everything else since then, but she's still worth it. I need to tell her that more often.

About two years later, after the birth of our first son, I was sitting in Langley, CIA headquarters, with a friend who worked for Security. He asked me what had ever come of the "conditional" part of our marriage, and whether I had been granted final approval. I answered that I had not yet heard a word. So he picked up the phone and dialed a contact in another section—probably the government Bureau of Conditional Approval for Goofy Guys Who Insist on Marrying Foreigners—to learn the outcome. The government has lots of bureaus, which is why it is called a bureaucracy.

Vic: "Hello. Can you tell me the status of B. D.'s marriage?"

Security: "Let me check. Yes, got his file right here . . . he was fired a year and half ago."

Vic (with a shocked look on his face): "Well, that's funny, because he's sitting right here next to me and has a badge on."

Yes, Security had indeed decided to fire me, probably based upon someone's resentment that I had flown home to get married without approval. I know of no other reason and was never given an explanation. But that's life in the government. All I knew at the time was that I had been terminated and they had neglected to tell anyone, including me. And the Agency, at least some offices, wasn't aware that I had continued working there for two years.

Things eventually worked out, and the CIA decided to keep me. That was more than a quarter century ago that my inner-Tarzan won that argument and I made the long walk around the swimming pool on the Dark Continent and found my Jane. That was a quarter century ago that I wouldn't take no for an answer—not from my wife (in the beginning), not from her mother, not from the Consulate Officer, not from family and friends, and not from all those supervisors at the CIA. There were lots and lots of no's.

But that one *oui* from a precious young lady made it all worth it.

Girls, tell him no a few times, before a yes. Make him work, to see if he will sacrifice, and find out if he is persistent. Test him for determination. If he gives his all to hold on to you while you are dating, through "thick and thin," then there is a good chance that he will never let go. I certainly won't.

NOTES

1. Edgar Rice Burroughs, *Tarzan of the Apes* (Chicago: A. C. McClurg & Co., 1914), 244.

11

Levels of Alertness

S ome people are naturally alert. Others . . . not so much. I sometimes feel that I'm not particularly attentive, especially not with details. I actually hate details, so I've compensated over the years by making lists, especially "to do" lists. I even had "not to do" lists, like many young men.

I couldn't rely on "to do" lists in the CIA, at least not lists with anything classified written on them. Imagine being stopped at a road block, and the police officer finding your list, reading, "Things to do during my secret meeting with Ivan: 1) make sure no one is following me, 2) pay him lots of money for spying, 3) tell him to be careful on his way back to the Defense Ministry, 4) avoid surveillance on the way home, and 5) pick up milk and eggs at the grocery store."

People operate at various levels of awareness during their everyday activities. And they often live or die depending on the level of awareness in which they are operating. When drivers are not alert, they can fall asleep at the wheel and kill themselves and others. Golfers hit others with their golf balls. Football players are blindsided by rampaging linebackers. Hunters shoot other hunters. Kids step on dresses.

There's a joke about a cowboy who walks up to a deer hunter who has just made a kill. The hunter is startled and yells at the cowboy, "Hey, get away from my deer!" The cowboy replies, "Okay, okay, relax! Can I at least get my saddle?"

Soldiers need to be alert and aware of their surroundings. I once traveled to Africa to conduct training for their military. We were scheduled to begin firearms training the following week and wanted to inspect their firing range. When we arrived, we asked our African hosts what was located on the other side of the berm, behind the targets. They replied that they did not know, so we walked over the hill, to see what we could see. And there, right in the line of fire, was an elementary school. That showed a lack of awareness on their part.

On the last day of our firearms training, it began to rain, and the students asked if they could place the remaining ammunition in the back of our vehicle to take to their armory. After a short classroom session, we left the base with the now-forgotten ammunition still in the trunk. Later that night, and after dinner at a restaurant, we were driving back to our hotel and were stopped by soldiers at a roadblock. One of them asked my colleague, who was driving, to open the trunk. When he did, we were quickly surrounded by nervous, young soldiers, cocking their assault rifles and pointing them at our heads.

Military coups in most African countries are prevented by a harsh, often brutal response to any hint of rebellion. In many African countries, it's illegal to have a single bullet. We had a trunk full of cases—thousands of rounds—of ammunition. Often, in those situations, young soldiers will shoot first and ask questions later, as they say.

Fortunately, they did not shoot. It took hours, but we were able to convince them that we were not mercenaries that had infiltrated to overthrow their government. At around 3:00 a.m., we were released. That mistake, which could have been a deadly one, showed a lack of awareness on our part.

Being alert is key. While attending a firearms course taught at Gunsite, Arizona, I learned of a simple awareness coding system differentiated by colors: white, yellow, orange, and red. These colors effectively delineate the various levels of alertness in the human psychology:

White: a person in condition White is basically "asleep at the wheel." She's too relaxed and oblivious to her surroundings. She's distracted, engrossed in a text message, or daydreaming. White means that she will walk into a telephone pole, step in a ditch, or cross the tracks in front of a moving train, she is so clueless. White means that a predator could kidnap her whenever and wherever he would like (or force himself inside her front door, as she enters). He can even surveil her for days, or weeks, and know everything about her: where she likes to eat out, where she shops, where she studies, where she lives, and whom she is dating. She is easy pickings. This is obviously not a condition where a young lady should be living, mentally.

Yellow: A young lady in condition Yellow is at a heightened level of awareness. She's relaxed but alert. She's not worried, afraid, nor paranoid because she's alert. She's aware of what is going on around her, of other shoppers in her vicinity, pedestrians on the street, passengers on her bus or subway car, other students in the library, people in the park. She's calm but casually notices who glances at her in a hotel lobby, if someone is watching her, or who is edging closer to her in a nightclub. She will notice anyone that is following her by using instinctive counter-surveillance techniques (more later) and by being aware of people near her, especially their demeanor. This is the recommended, minimum level at which a young lady should operate until, of course, a threat causes her to move to orange.

Orange: Condition Orange indicates that she has seen something specific that concerns her—she has now identified a potential threat. For example, she has confirmed that a man has been following her through the library, on several floors or through several sections, or is approaching her near the restrooms of a restaurant. Maybe a Gweebi, with whom she mistakenly went on a date (yes, she missed the warning signs during vetting, testing, and eliciting) has told her that he will not take her home—contrary to her wishes and requests—and insists on driving her up into the mountains to "talk things out." She tells him to take her home now. Immediately. Depending upon his response, she is now ready for condition Red and the flight or fight decision.

Red: At this point, she's going to choose one or the other—flight or fight—which means that she'll either try to escape or fight him. The man who followed her in the library has approached her vehicle in the parking lot and is trying to grab her or push her in the car. She either struggles to escape and run or punches him in the face or shoots him. She screams for help from friends, restaurant staff, or anyone. She draws attention to her situation. The man who has backed her against the wall or tried to pull her out the back door of the restaurant? She resists, giving him a knee to the crotch, and she yells for help. The unfortunate date with a Gweebi who has now turned sexual predator? She gets out of his car when he stops at the next traffic signal or she yells at him to let her out and warns that she will call the police. And she hits the speed dial on her phone to call her dad, brother, or 911.

Some might argue that a young woman can't walk around paranoid all of the time, reasoning that there are times she can let down her guard: she might live in a small town or she's safe at school, with relatives, or at church. I agree; a young woman should not live life being paranoid. Not everyone is out to get her.

But she should live life in condition Yellow, which is a comfortable and safe condition, leading a less paranoid life. She should not feel paranoid, because she's confident and proud that she's taking care of herself. She should not feel scared because she is prepared.

But hey, maybe she can be in condition White at church. As I write this, I see a headline on CNN, "Preacher accused of 59 counts of molesting girls in Minnesota": Victor Barnard allegedly convinced his church congregants to allow their daughters to join a church camp. Now, he's on the run, charged with sexually assaulting two of the girls.[1]

Yes, unfortunately, we live in a world where young girls should be in condition Yellow all of the time, even at church.

And for parents who might feel like they do not want to live life being "paranoid," it's not hard to find more scary stories. As I write this, I just finished reading another article: "Mom and Dad Wondered Why Their Daughter, 13, Was Getting So Many 'Friend' Requests—When They Learned the Truth, They Called Police." The article reads, "The mother . . . told authorities she was concerned about the spike in 'friend requests' that her young teenage daughter was receiving, so she did some parental investigating. A scan of the child's tablet revealed she was 'exchanging nude photos of herself with teenage boys.'"[2]

Parents should also live in condition Yellow. Always.

If being self-aware is the first step to self-protection, then awareness of surroundings and others is next. Condition Yellow, and awareness, keeps a gazelle alive in the Serengeti and a girl safe in her world. Girls and parents, be alert like a gazelle.

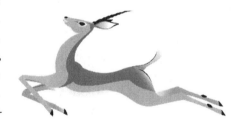

NOTES

1. Steve Almsay and Carman Hassan, "Preacher Accused of 59 Counts of Molesting Girls in Minnesota," April 14, 2014, http://www.cnn.com/2014/04/17/justice/minnesota-preacher-manhunt/.

2. Mike Opelka, "Mom and Dad Wondered Why Their Daughter, 13, Was Getting So Many 'Friend' Requests—When They Learned the Truth, They Called Police," April 17, 2014, http://www.theblaze.com/stories/2014/08/22/mom-and-dad-wondered-why-their-daughter-13-was-getting-so-many-friend-requests-when-they-learned-the-truth-they-called-police/.

12

Countersurveillance

Boys will be boys. Boys will also be boys who enjoy watching girls. My ten-year-old son and I were driving home recently when he noticed our neighbor's granddaughters, around his age, playing in their front yard. As he was watching them, intently, I playfully kidded, "Don't be looking at all those pretty girls!"

He looked up at me with a puzzled look on his face and asked, "Why not?"

Most young women are probably fine with nice young men watching them. Otherwise, why all that time in front of the mirror? But they obviously don't want attention from bad men. And they especially don't want attention from sexual predators.

Countersurveillance refers to measures that a woman can take to be aware of others watching or following her. She can use countersurveillance to detect, avoid, or thwart surveillance, whether it be surveillance by a hostile intelligence organization, a terrorist group, or a sexual predator.

Countersurveillance measures in espionage or law enforcement involve moving in certain ways to draw out a surveillant and to expose him. A person might work to expose surveillants who are watching her during an operation or even during her commute to and from work.

Countersurveillance measures to detect surveillance by a terrorist group are more intense because they involve armed individuals, possibly an entire assault team. These forces will also project an image of a hard target, an effective deterrent, which can often dissuade a potential attacker and prevent an attack before it ever takes shape.

Countersurveillance measures can also be employed to thwart a predatory young man or a stalker before a situation escalates. A woman can identify a stalker and recognize his bad behavior early on. And isn't it so much better to detect the creep and stop him in his tracks before he evolves, or devolves, into a stalker?

POWERS OF OBSERVATION

Countersurveillance can be boiled down to a few words: observation over time and distance.

Let's start with observation. My favorite word in the Greek language is παρατηρητικότητα (*paratiritikotita*), which means "powers of observation." Powers of observation refers to the ability to be conscious of your surroundings and to identify details and actions. In terms of countersurveillance, it is the ability to see and identify someone who is watching or following you and who might be a threat by his appearance, features, clothing, or vehicle.

Most women are natural observers. My wife has an inherent ability to identify vehicles. She might not know the make and model, but she can connect most owners in our neighborhood to their vehicles and many others around town. She is instinctively observant, as are most women.

My wife is also a great observer of people. I often brought her along to diplomatic functions when I was fishing for potential sources, or spies. And she is sociable; in fact, she enjoys a party more than most. She enjoys getting to know new people, and she was actually a lot better at it than I was. At a party, I'm much more comfortable sitting on the edge of the room, observing others mingle, preferably finding one good friend with whom I can discuss politics or sports and tell jokes. My wife, on the other hand, prefers being in the mix.

At most gatherings, my wife and I would split up in order to cover more ground. Invariably, I would return a short while later to find her visiting amiably with another woman, possibly the spouse of a Russian diplomat or high-ranking Asian. I would then just wait by her side until the husband came looking for his wife. My wife should have been on the CIA's payroll.

After the parties, my wife could tell me the names of diplomats she met, what they were wearing, what others were wearing, what people said (advice to men: never argue with a woman about what was said in a conversation!), even who was attracted to whom or who was mad at whom. She could tell all this by their conversations, actions, and even furtive glances. Remember, women can carry on a whole conversation without saying a word.

My wife has excellent παρατηρητικότητα. And if a young lady wants to be good at "counter-creep-surveillance," then she must tap into this inherent ability that women have.

How are your observations skills?

What color was Tammy's dress, in the first chapter?
What is the hairstyle of the little girl holding flowers, in chapter 2?
How many darts are in the target, in chapter 3?

How were your observation skills? And your recollection?

Once a young lady has tapped into her παρατηρητικότητα, she can then use a few spy techniques:

1. Time, distance, with multiple sightings. For a young lady to conclude that she's being watched, she must see the same person several times, separated by time and distance.

For example, if a young lady sees a man on the cereal aisle of the grocery store, and again in produce a few minutes later, the sequence of events is not significant enough to merit suspicion. If a young lady sees a man in a shoe store in the shopping mall, and again ten minutes later purchasing a drink three stores down, that's also minimal time and minimal distance. The situation is probably not alarming.

If, however, she notices a young man in the next aisle of a music store perusing music CDs, and again in Macey's a half hour later, looking at shoes and possibly looking her way, and then at the other end of the mall in Cheesecake Factory an hour later, she has reason to be concerned and will raise her level of alertness to Orange. She has seen him over a period of time, in various locations a distance apart, and multiple times—check, check, and check.

I feel that these concepts of time and distance may be compressed in a department store, depending on the number of sightings, but also taking into consideration the congested nature of such a store. A young lady might notice someone next to her in Sporting Goods, then in the Garden section, and again in Electronics. At this point, the young lady should make an obvious move through the store, attempting to provoke a reaction from the potential surveillant: walk to Eyewear, over to Pharmacy, then to Women's Clothes, for example. It will become readily apparent if the man is following her.

2. Zigzag routes. As I've already mentioned, most people are creatures of habit. People put on each pant leg in the same order, socks and shoes in the same way, even brush their teeth in the same sequence. People drive to and from work at the same time of the day using the same route and buy their coffee at the same shop. It is all about convenience and routine. Unfortunately, convenience gets people kidnapped or killed in dangerous areas. And convenience renders young women vulnerable.

By merely walking a somewhat zigzag route through a department store, a young woman is much more likely to spot someone following her. For example, walking all the way down one wall of the store then turning left at the end and walking down the next wall to the Electronics section will require a predator to make only one turn while following you. Going through the middle of the store, however, then making several turns along different aisles (like a stair pattern) forces the predator to take several turns to follow her and exposes him to detection. The girl can casually see behind her at every turn.

The same can be done with driving. Take a few turns here and there rather than beelining to a destination. And watch in your rearview mirror to notice if another vehicle is making the same turns with you. It is much easier to spot a predator who has taken turn after turn with you, either through a park, neighborhood, or department store, or while driving, than when you travel along a straight line. Don't be an easy target. Don't make it easy for someone to follow you.

There are hilarious movies that show actors sprinting through train stations, jumping tracks, and racing their vehicles through alleys to escape surveillance. This is usually unnecessary, unless you're running for your life. Usually subtle but deliberate movements can clarify a situation.

3. Reversals. A reversal refers to your turning—reversing—in the direction from which you had just come, either on the same aisle, road, path, or a parallel path, where you are able to clearly see someone behind you.

Reversals might include your looking at the person in the eye and letting him know that you are aware he is behind you. If he's someone with no evil intent, then his demeanor will show that, and he will walk on by and maybe even smile at you. If the person is following you, however, it could be readily apparent by watching his facial expression and his demeanor as he looks away, nervously glances at you, or exhibits some uncomfortable behavior.

A reversal can be carried out in a store aisle, a shopping mall hallway (on the way to the restrooms), or while driving (U-turn).

While working in Europe, I going to a meeting and was climbing the steps from the subway station. When I arrived at the top, I noticed that I had emerged on the wrong side of the street (many stations have multiple exits/entrances to accommodate pedestrians). When I turned back to descend, I noticed a man following behind me as he was just beginning to climb the stairs. When he saw me turn and start toward him, he looked surprised, turned around, and hurried away from me. Was he just startled to see a large man turn and come back toward him? Was he a member of an intelligence agency following me? I don't know, but it was suspicious. Had I seen him again, I could've confirmed that he was following me. This innocent, unintentional reversal had possibly exposed a surveillant.

4. Chokepoints. A young woman should be aware of points along a route—whether walking or driving—where she is forced to go through a "bottleneck," or route that allows only one way to pass, such as a footbridge over a river connecting one area of a city to another. For example, department stores often allow only one or two exits. A predator might not have to follow a young lady through a store and will decide to wait near the exit for her to return to her car. Be extra vigilant at chokepoints.

5. Mirrors, mirrors on the wall. A woman can find ways to magnify her field of vision without showing that she is wary (which might cause a stalker to pull back even further and be increasingly cautious and harder to detect). There are mirrors everywhere. Walls of shopping malls, high-rises, and stores are covered with mirrors. And it's easy to approach a mirror and see everyone that is behind you: the lady with the red blouse, the two teenagers, the blond man with blue T-shirt and jeans.

A young woman might stop at a sunglasses kiosk to shop for sunglasses. There's a mirror on the counter, so she glances at other shoppers while she tries on a pair: the mother pushing a stroller, the children running in the indoor playground, the blond man wearing a blue T-shirt and jeans. She then enters Walgreens and lingers near the entrance, perusing books, and looks across the top of the aisle, through the window, noticing people approaching the front door: a woman in a tie-dye sarong, a man in a gray suit, two older ladies in dresses, and . . . a blond man with a blue T-shirt and jeans. She now realizes that the man seems to be following her, thanks to her powers of observation and help from mirrors and windows.

A trained surveillant would most likely notice a young lady using mirrors or windows. Most creeps, on the other hand, aren't trained, and aren't as observant as you.

6. Check his demeanor: Like the man exiting the subway station, predators, stalkers, or surveillants will often exhibit behaviors that a target can detect and identify as suspicious. A young woman can sometimes see a correlation between her movements and those of a predator: he might enter a bookstore right after her, he stops perusing books when she does, he finishes his coffee soon after her, he moves at the same time and departs at the same time.

She might also notice that he will not make eye contact, other than furtive glances, while walking past him through a row of books in the library. His body language will also reveal his true intent: sudden stops, wandering, lack of any real purpose in his movements. His demeanor will reveal him.

7. Surveillance Detection Route (SDRs): In the world of espionage, an SDR is used to detect surveillance, as the term implies. An officer or someone concerned about being targeted may design a route to draw out and identify surveillance by visiting various stores or areas, hoping to expose members of a hostile surveillance. A stationary surveillant (static surveillance) sitting in a cafe by a park is much more difficult to detect than someone who is being forced to move (mobile surveillance) and forced to react to the movements of the target, constantly trying to keep up with and not lose her— especially an observant, vigilant woman.

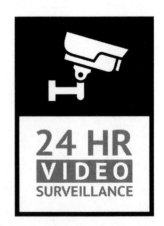

If a young lady senses that someone is following her, even if it is just a feeling, she might make a few stops on her way to work: she first pulls into a McDonald's drive-through for a morning egg biscuit (which is much tastier than an Egg McMuffin, as everyone knows!), and notices the cars in her vicinity: a blue Toyota Prius with female driver and male passenger behind her, a white Camaro two vehicles back, a maroon Ford F-150 pickup truck with male driver pulling in a parking space across the street, and a white minivan with kids parked on the street. She next goes to a gas station and, while filling her tank, casually scans the area: a green BMW, a blue Dodge Ram pickup, and a maroon Ford F-150 with male driver—who she now sees has black hair and goatee.

She then heads to Speedy Dry-cleaning, located five miles away, picks up her clothes, and is again observant as she exits and approaches her vehicle: there is a green mini-Cooper with female driver, a red Toyota Tundra, other parked vehicles with no drivers, and . . . a maroon Ford F-150 pick-up truck with a male driver, the same man with black hair and goatee. She then drives through a shopping district, takes a few turns, and notices the same maroon F-150 behind her, taking the same turns.

She now has a situation that meets the criteria for time, distance, multiple sightings. At the stoplight, she writes down his license plate number and as complete a description of the driver and vehicle as she can. She hits her speed dial to contact her father, brother, or 911. If she decides to contact the police, she is able to provide enough information to proceed with an investigation.

All young women should be "countersurveillants" by nature, always aware of their surroundings and of people in their vicinity and be able to detect someone following them, identifying those with bad intentions. Small, seemingly insignificant acts, which become habits, can make the difference between life and death: noticing a new vehicle in your apartment complex, one that you have not seen in the past; noticing who is in line with you in the checkout; seeing who is pumping gas in a vehicle next to you at the 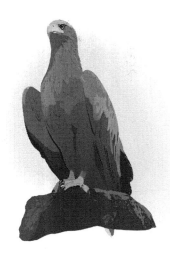 gas station; scanning the parking lot as you walk toward your car in the parking lot; maybe spotting a man lingering near vehicles. Small acts can be the difference between being kidnapped and being safe.

Girls need to be observant, to surveil, and to watch like a hawk.

1. Notice others over time and distance. Be observant.
2. Use zigzag routes while walking through stores or driving.
3. Use natural reversals.
4. Be extra alert at chokepoints.
5. Casually use mirrors and windows.
6. Notice his demeanor.
7. Notice correlations between your movements and another's, and practice an SDR (surveillance detection route).

13

Counterfeits

Counterfeit money is often hard to spot, even for an expert. Counterfeit bonds, checks, coupons, antiques, and certificates are equally deceiving. They all appear deceptively real or authentic.

There is even counterfeit clothing, such as shoes, shirts, and neckties. I was in Seoul, South Korea, for a short period of time during the late 1980s. In the evenings, after work hours, I sometimes shopped in a suburb called Itawon, which is known for counterfeit merchandise. As I was looking through neckties in a small shop, I noticed a tag attached to one that read, "mung ju silk." I was curious, so I showed the tag to the storekeeper and asked what it meant in English. She looked left and then right—rather secretly—before she whispered, in a heavy accent, "poly-es-tah."

There are even counterfeit cures, such as the Virgin Cleansing Myth. Men all over Africa who suffer from the HIV infection are persuaded by "traditional healers" that they can be healed by having sex with a virgin girl. The men are desperate and want to believe, and, in their desperation, pass HIV to untold numbers of young women around the continent.

I wonder if God has reserved a special place in hell for the first man who came up with the Virgin Cleansing Myth.

Journalist Thomas C. Frohlich wrote, "Because the recession placed people under considerable financial pressure, it may have made them easier targets for fraud." He quotes John M. Simpson, consumer advocate at Consumer Watchdog, who said, "If you're in debt, you're desperate, and so you might try anything." Frohlich continued, "Highly indebted individuals may be more likely to suspend their disbelief and fall victim to a scam . . . they may even be desperate enough to engage in fraud themselves."[1]

That is really what it boils down to—victims suspending disbelief. When people are vulnerable—in financial debt or ill—they will convince themselves that something is true when it's not, that a cure works when it does not, and that someone is honest, when he is not. When a woman is lonely, in financial trouble, or otherwise vulnerable, she may fall victim to a scheme (or a man) she might otherwise see as a fraud.

While most of us would consider a con man to be rather repulsive, they can be charming and friendly and can even be fun to watch. I witnessed a modern-day con man working his magic a few years ago. He was a traveling salesman from Arizona, a modern-day carpetbagger making his monthly rounds. He had come through our town to visit a friend of mine and other customers, or "suckers," to peddle monthly allotments of enzymes, supplements, and cures (although most are careful to avoid saying that word) to guard against parasites, blood ailments, and other diseases.

When we were introduced, he grasped my hand in both of his. I have to say, I don't trust a man who does that. I especially don't trust traveling salesmen peddling enzymes and other miracle cures who also present me with the dreaded, double-handshake. As he held my hand, he looked me over, sized me up, and quickly diagnosed that I was also suffering from infirmities, blood issues, and parasites.

BELIEF AND SUSPENDING DISBELIEF

As Frolich noted, desperate, suffering individuals willingly suspend disbelief, or believe notions that are not rational. That is one reason we go to the cinema to watch a movie: we suspend disbelief while accepting the notion that there are blue people with tails on another planet who fly around on multicolored dinosaur birds, who sometimes attack helicopters funded by evil corporations searching for "unobtanium." We suspend disbelief all the time in movie theaters, going along for the experience or "ride." But at least we leave the theater after the movie with our wallets intact (other than the nine dollar price of admission).

However, when we suspend disbelief in other venues, such as on the Internet, on the street, in a train station, or in a relationship, we stand to lose more. We can lose a whole wallet, our home, our pride, or even our heart.

In reality, we need to maintain a healthy dose of disbelief, or skepticism.

DETECTING COUNTERFEIT MEN

Women need to be alert for counterfeit men—men who try to appear deceptively real or authentic. She must listen to every word that comes out of a man's mouth, and believe half of it. When she hears a man say something that causes her spy skills to tingle or that just doesn't sound right, she should ask herself: "What the . . . ? Why did he say that? Does he expect me to believe that?"

She should pause and consider carefully when a young man says something like,

- "Oh, you just don't want to ride on my motorcycle because you're chicken."
- "Yeah, your parents probably wouldn't let you go on a cruise with me anyway."
- "Well, you're probably too young to be out this late. Past your bedtime?"
- "You dress like a pioneer woman! Are you too shy to show a little skin?"
- "I'm feeling sad and lonely. I just need someone to hold me."
- "If you really do love me, why not prove it with more affection?"
- "Did it hurt, when you fell from heaven?"
- "Are you Jamaican? Because Jamaican me crazy . . ."

LOCK YOUR HEART

A predator on the streets of New York might only steal a young lady's money. A used car salesman might reduce her bank account. But a con-man predator in a dating situation will read a young lady like a book, play her like a violin, and then drop her like a rock. He will also steal her heart in the process and not return it in the same condition.

How many women have been duped into abusive relationships, sexual assault, rape, or murder, based largely on their belief in what a man told her? That would be quite a statistic—maybe a huge, unknowable number.

Do not let belief be the key that unlocks your heart. Do not open your heart to a young man too quickly, and especially not based on your belief in what he says. Do not have faith in men whom you do not know, or even someone you do know but have not yet vetted and tested. Be wary of young men who seem too good to be true.

NOTES

1. Thomas C. Frohlich, "Top States with the Most Fraud Complaints," *USA Today*, March 8, 2014.

14
Lies and Disguise

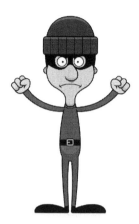

When you really think about it, men and books have a lot in common. Both can be fat or thin, well cared for or worn. Some are leather-bound. Some are gilded, while others are faded or dog-eared with broken backs. They both wear jackets and sometimes use covers. They come in all shapes, sizes, and visible conditions, none of which reveals the inner quality. Like the old saying, "never judge a book by its cover."

Interestingly, an author will use a cover for his book just as a spy will choose a cover for his job. And he will use a disguise to aid in enhancing his cover and his appearance. He uses the disguise to take on an identity or persona. This persona can be a character or social facade that he can adopt at different times or in various situations.

In the CIA, I took on an alias, or cover, to facilitate meeting people from various backgrounds under various circumstances. And I used multiple disguises over the years: fake mustaches, collodion scars, clear lens glasses, hats, wigs, and more.

I was just employing another art: the art of disguise.

Unfortunately for women, bad men are artful in the use of disguises to change their persona, or more accurately, to mask their true persona. A man who is rotten to the core can still disguise himself nicely on the outside. He can wear expensive clothes, fix his hair and teeth, and sprinkle himself with luxurious cologne.

Most men are convinced that cologne works best of all, probably due to the influence of advertising. A man knows that if he smells nice, if he douses himself with enough body spray, beautiful angels will literally fall from the sky and surround him. Another cologne claims to render even a robot irresistible to beautiful women. When I was young, it was Hai Karate, a budget aftershave that was sold with an instruction booklet on how to defend oneself from swarms of women who were uncontrollably attracted to the smell.

I tried it and was ready to defend myself from all the attractive women. Alas, it didn't work for me. I still believe that there must be some truth behind the campaigns, or manufacturers and advertisers wouldn't keep pushing the notion that women can be manipulated by smells. So men will continue to try it, just to see if women attack!

But are women that easily manipulated by their senses? By what they hear, what they see, and even by what they smell?

Ladies, look at the following photographs and ask yourself, "which one of these handsome devils would I date, judging by his appearance alone?"

TED BUNDY

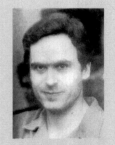

This good-looking man was a convicted serial killer. He confessed to killing thirty people in several states during the late 1970s. Ted Bundy was considered intelligent, charming, and handsome.

PHILIP MARKOFF

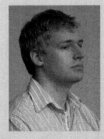

Philip Markoff was a medical student who was charged with murder and armed robbery, until he committed suicide. He was called the Craigslist Killer because he allegedly met his victims through ads on Craigslist.

SCOTT PETERSON

Scott Peterson is on death row for the murder of his wife and her unborn son in 2002. Judging by his appearance alone, you might not think that someone could be that vicious.

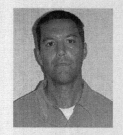

JORAN VAN DER SLOOT

Joran Van der Sloot is a Dutch citizen and convicted murderer. He is currently serving twenty-eight years for the murder of Stephany Ramirez in 2010, in Lima, Peru. He is also suspected in the murder of an American teenager, Natalee Holloway.

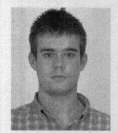

HERMAN WEBSTER MUDGETT

Herman Webster Mudgett, also known as Dr. Henry Howard Holmes, one of the first reported serial killers in America, confessed to killing at least thirty people (possibly as many as two hundred). Most of his victims were females.

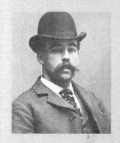

I suppose that I could go on and list more recent Casanova criminals, or go back further in time, as far back as Cain in the Old Testament. Cain was probably tall, dark, and handsome and might have smelled good too.

But I do not want this to be a dark downer of a book. I just want to warn women, young and old, to not be fooled by a man's (or woman's), appearance, charm, smell, or persona. I want women to open their eyes to a truth—that they cannot just see with their eyes or their nose. To quote the Little Prince, "The essential is invisible to the eye."[1]

A woman needs to be aware that a man can use a disguise to mask who he really is. He will use a disguise to deceive. And there are many, many types of disguises, some not as obvious as a nice suit or cologne.

The Internet can actually serve as an effective disguise for a man, another world where he can hide his true self and his true intentions.

He can use it to exaggerate or obfuscate his life or accomplishments and even take on someone else's identity. So women should be extra vigilant when communicating with someone over the Internet, keeping in mind that maybe nothing he posts or tweets is true. If she is in contact with someone via social media, she should look for inconsistencies, "red flags," or "whiffs" (remember how to spot a liar, in Chapter 6) that he is hiding something, acting like someone he is not, or straight-up lying. She can also call upon her friends, her "sources," to help her vet someone via Facebook, Twitter, or other social media to find out if he acts or communicates differently with others than he does with her. If she suspects something, she should trust her instincts.

Predators, especially, use the Internet to disguise their attempts to target their victims, particularly the youth. According to Microsoft Safety and Security Center, they will do the following:[2]

- Find kids through social networking, blogs, chat rooms, instant messaging, email, discussion boards, and other websites.
- Seduce their targets through attention, affection, kindness, and even gifts.
- Know the latest music and hobbies likely to interest kids.
- Listen to and sympathize with kids' problems.
- Try to ease young people's inhibitions by gradually introducing sexual content into their conversation or by showing them sexually explicit material.
- Might also evaluate the kids they meet online for future face-to-face contact.

The Internet can be a sex offender's "disguise." A young woman might believe that she is chatting with another fifteen-year-old male or female, when in fact she is being targeted by a fifty-five-year-old predator. Women need to be aware that they can be fooled by a predator's appearance in person or by his profile on the Internet.

It happened to Manti Te'o, the Notre Dame football star. It also happened to six women at Brigham Young University. These six women were scammed by the same individual. Each was in a "romantic" online relationship with an individual they thought was a handsome blonde man named Hunter. In fact, their online relationships weren't with Hunter at all, but with another female who had stolen his identity and then posed as a male. One of the victims noted, "I think we wouldn't expect this kind of thing to happen. . . . Your initial reaction when you're talking to someone isn't 'Oh, they're probably sending me pictures of someone else and lying to me about who they are.'"[3]

A girl must ask herself: Could this person be lying? Could this be a scam? Who is really behind the profile? Who is behind the mask?

My intention is not to make a young lady afraid to use the Internet. But she must be aware of the dangers of disguised predators on the Internet. How can she minimize the risk of being a victim? Here are a few, life-saving suggestions excerpted from a list prepared by Microsoft:

- Use family settings on the computer.
- Follow age limits on social networking websites.
- Keep the Internet-connected computer in a common area of the house.
- Never download images from an unknown source—they could be sexually explicit.
- Choose a gender-neutral screen name that does not contain sexually suggestive words or reveal personal information.
- Never reveal personal information about yourself (including age and gender) or information about your family to anyone online.
- Stop any email communication, instant messaging conversations, or chats if anyone starts to ask questions that are too personal or sexually suggestive.
- Post a family agreement near the computer to remind you to protect your privacy on the Internet.[4]

Ladies, use your spy skills to see through a man's disguise, to see behind his mask, and to see his true identity and persona. Do not be fooled by the gold gilding, the charm, the tall-dark-and-handsomeness, or the seductive scent of his Hai Karate. Look beyond the cover.

Do not be fooled by someone's appearance when meeting him in person and especially not on the Internet. Do not judge a book, or young man, by his cover.

1. Look beyond the disguise.
2. Don't judge a book by its cover.
3. Be wary when using the Internet.

NOTES

1. Antoine de St. Exupéry, *Le Petit Prince* (New York: Harcourt, 2001).

2. Microsoft.com, Safety and Security Centre, Family Safety, "Online predators: Help minimize the risk," https://www.microsoft.com/en-gb/security/family-safety/predators.aspx.

3. Jenna Koford and Bret Henkel, "BYU Women victimized by 'catfish' relationship deception," *The Digital Universe*, March 17, 2015.

4. Microsoft.com, Safety and Security Centre, Family Safety.

Photo of Ted Bundy courtesy of State Archives of Florida, Florida Memory.

15

Break the Chain

> "Over 13 percent of women in college have reported
> being a victim of stalking during the school year, and
> one out of every five college women has reported being
> sexually assaulted. It is simple to talk about statistics.
> It is more difficult to remember that each number is a
> victim and represents a daughter, a sister or a friend."[1]
>
> **—US Rep. Gwen Moore**

Sexual predators, or assailants of any type, use the same targeting techniques. They engage in tedious planning, just like my wife's disgusting uncle (see page 18). They often follow a "chain of attack": target selection, surveillance, final target confirmation, more surveillance, ambush site selection, deployment, and attack. An assailant will select a target based upon value, vulnerabilities, and whether the intended victim is a soft or hard target—meaning he wants to be successful and escape unharmed. And he prefers a target with vulnerabilities.

To find vulnerabilities, a predator will watch the target to confirm her value, habits, and routes used during the daily routine. Bank officials have been assassinated driving home from the office because they always used the same bridges (chokepoint) at the same times. A government official in Latin America was assassinated as he arrived at his mistress's home. His attackers knew where he was going to be and when he would arrive because he regularly visited her at her home: same time, same place.

Once an assailant has selected a target and has conducted preliminary surveillance, he will draw an X, figuratively, at the spot where he will conduct the ambush. This is where he wants the target to be. Additional surveillance confirms when he wants her there so he doesn't have to linger too long at the attack site. For example, he knows that the target arrives at her gym every day at 8:30 a.m. He can then show up at 8:15 and be there for only a short period of time—too short a time to draw attention or arouse suspicion from witnesses who could alert the police and stop the attack. For assailants and predators, the when and where is key.

We have discussed many ways to avoid becoming a victim. Many ideas are strategic solutions to the problem. There are also tactical solutions.

Let's talk about a few:

1. Vary your times, routes, and donkeys! Staying off the attacker's X is a matter of you not being where he wants you to be when he wants you to be there. And this can be accomplished by changing where you go and when you go there.

There are usually myriad ways to walk or drive from any two points, such as from your apartment to your college class. So instead of walking to class at Columbia University the same way at the same time, every day, every evening (like a creature of habit), a young woman can change her route: she can walk down 113th instead of 114th street and up Amsterdam instead of Broadway. And instead of leaving her apartment at 7:45 each morning for her 8:00 class, she can depart her home at 7:00 from time to time and go to the library to study or leave at 6:30 to work out at the gym.

Since we are all creatures of habit, this might be difficult to do. People love routine. We love to know that we can walk up Broadway because it takes exactly the same amount of time every day and there is a nice sidewalk and a place that sells the most delicious bagels along the way. Habits and routine are hard to break because we love convenience and routine.

People love routine. Vulnerable people especially love routine. And predators love vulnerable people who love their routine.

I found myself in bad places when I worked for the CIA, and I wonder sometimes that maybe I am still here, alive on this planet earth, because of some little thing that I did right. Maybe it was a precaution that I took. Maybe I went to work via a different route one day—the same day that assailants had planned to kill me. Maybe I left home a little earlier than usual and they missed me. Maybe it was also luck. Maybe I was lucky that someone didn't plant explosives in the donkey that I slapped on the side of the road when I drove by one morning in a Humvee with my National Guard friends.

But we also make our own luck. And maybe it was because they didn't know where I was or when I was going to drive by or which donkey I was going to slap. So vary your times, routes, and donkeys.

Of course, there are some areas that a young lady or young man should stay away from at all times. Be aware of high-crime neighborhoods or even shopping areas that should be avoided altogether.

2. Dress the part. Some people dress to attract attention. Others, like my older son, don't care at all about clothes and grab whatever is clean (maybe) and close at hand. But even those ladies who admittedly don't care about clothes, whether they blend or attract attention, are still doing one or the other. Not making a choice is a choice.

Tourists are advised to dress like locals to blend in and to not advertise that they are foreigners and thus attract pickpockets, or worse. Intelligence officers dress in certain ways to camouflage, to disguise, to confuse, and to blend. Women have the same choices: blend or attract, camouflage or highlight, or even to disguise and confuse.

Men are going to always notice what women are wearing, ever since Eve first put clothes on. And women are going to attract men, good and bad, based on what they are wearing. A woman walking across campus in a bikini top and short shorts is going to turn heads, including a bad man's head. The same woman walking across in pants or an attractive dress may still turn heads, but science (and not merely male chauvinism) tells us one is going to attract more attention than the other. Again, I would never suggest that it's the woman's fault if she's targeted or assaulted. Nothing justifies an assault, stalking, or even unwanted approaches. But a woman can stay off certain men's radars simply by what she wears. She can dress for whatever part she wants in life's play.

3. Stop and wait before you get too close to something suspicious. No stalker, rapist, or run-of-the-mill creep targeting a woman will know exactly when she will arrive at a particular location. He is forced, therefore, to linger somewhere, whether it be a stairwell, a bus stop, or next to his parked car (any place where it's normal for someone to wait and easier to blend in). He will be forced to wait for her or for another victim who might be a softer target.

And while he's waiting, he's vulnerable. He will stand out and will be susceptible to detection. While he's waiting for her next to his X, maybe next to his van parked on the side of Broadway, he can appear nervous, awkward, unsure of himself, and unsure how to act. This is when an observant young lady can spot a predator before it is too late.

Let's say that a young student is walking home from the library somewhat late at night. She is walking up 115th street toward home and

notices a man approximately fifty yards away, standing next to his van—
with the door open.

What should she do? She could keep walking straight ahead, maybe
with her hand on her pepper spray. She doesn't want to show fear, right?
She feels like Katniss, of *The Hunger Games*. She's ready for anything.

But she doesn't have a bow and arrow like Katniss. What about just
stopping before she approaches the X? Why not stop and act like she is
talking on the telephone? What if she simply stops in her tracks, waits,
and watches? While she watches, she notices that he reaches into his open
car and picks up bags of groceries, turns toward the apartment building,
and walks inside. Smart Katniss knows at that point that he was not waiting for her and that he was merely carrying groceries inside his apartment.
So she continues on her way.

But what if, when she stops, the man looks at her and also stops what
he's doing (she notices correlation between her movements and his). He
doesn't appear to be engaged in anything purposeful and might even
appear confused or unsure what to do when he sees that she has stopped.
She then notices that he's glancing at her. At this point, the young lady,
who's still a safe distance away, turns around and walks in the other direction back to the library, or store, and calls a friend.

She might feel slightly embarrassed that she overreacted, but she also
feels safe and smart. And interestingly, she might not ever know that she
just saved her own life, just as I don't know if I ever saved mine.

If a young lady is driving home along a narrow, country road and
notices a car ahead, its trunk lid up, the driver and passenger outside,
what can she do? She can stop her vehicle well away from them and ensure
that her doors are locked. She can wait to see if it's an X. If it's not an X,
then she'll see the driver pull out the spare tire, the passenger pull out the
jack and lug wrench, and they'll start jacking up the car and continue
changing a flat tire and probably not notice her.

If they have bad intentions, however, they might look at her sitting
in her car, idling a safe distance away, and they'll wait, maybe fidgeting.
They won't know what to do because she has stopped well away from their
X and she's on the Y or Z, which throws off their plans completely. They
might just get in their car and drive away. But she might turn around in
a driveway and return in the other direction and drive to her destination
via another route, since she's not a creature of habit and can change her
route with ease.

If a young lady is walking down a back stairwell in a mall and hears whispering a few floors down at the entrance to the basement, what should she do? Should she proceed, courageous as Buffy the Vampire Slayer? Or can she wait at the top floor and listen? If they're waiting to assault someone, they'll stop talking and listen. If they're shoppers, however, then she'll hear them laugh at a joke or gather the belongings that they dropped on the stairs, and she'll watch them exit the building ahead of her.

If a young woman sees a man lingering at the entrance to her dorm as she approaches, what should she do? Should she proceed, like Xena the Princess Warrior, or can she wait for a minute across the street and watch him? Does he appear to have a purpose—like waiting for a girlfriend to exit—or is he looking around, shuffling, and acting suspicious? Does his demeanor indicate someone who is anxious to go on a first date or someone who is a predator?

She might wait for a minute and see his girlfriend run out the door and greet him with a kiss. Mystery solved. It took her only a minute to find out that he's not a criminal who is waiting for an unsuspecting lady to arrive and then force his way through the door with her and rape her in the stairwell.

If a young woman exits a theater and sees a man leave before her and glance over his shoulder, what should she do? Should she proceed because that's her favorite exit and she always takes it because it is near her car? Or she can just take the main exit and be a little inconvenienced.

She may never know that she just saved her life without having used her pepper spray (which she does have) or a flying Xena the Princess Warrior side-kick. But she will know that she is safe.

4. Don't be at the WPWTWP. Survival is often just a matter of avoiding those three things, those three mistakes: wrong place, wrong time, and wrong person. People are alive right now, talking with their family, driving a car, swimming, and eating dinner, because they avoided those six letters. Some people are dead, not talking, not driving, not swimming, and not eating, because they didn't avoid that deadly combination.

People follow many rules at the gun range when firing weapons: be aware of your target, don't point a gun at others, always treat a gun as if it's loaded, keep your finger off the trigger until you're ready to fire. These rules are meant to be redundant and overlapping. A shooter usually has to break several rules to cause an accident: she has to carelessly treat the gun as if it's unloaded, point it at someone, and then have her finger on the trigger. Accidents usually involve a whole series of mistakes.

Not all sexual assaults are brought on by mistakes. Some women make all the right decisions and still fall victim to predators. But a woman who breaks several safety rules will become only more vulnerable to an attack. She might drink one too many beers, decide to walk home alone, and then accept help from a stranger. The whole series of broken rules, of bad choices, eventually overwhelms her.

She might get into a vehicle with a young man who's drinking, show-ing off, or speeding. She might hop on the back of a motorcycle with a young man who likes to show how skillfully he can drive at night down a mountain road. She might not think twice about who is driving or how he is driving. She is too busy chatting, laughing, texting, and enjoying immortality.

I searched "young woman killed in car accident" online and found too many tragic news stories:

"Madisen Price was killed, while Delanie Price and Balstad were taken to Wyoming Medical Center . . . sister in a coma five days before her high school graduation . . . Wyoming Highway Patrol said both drinking and speed may have been involved."[2]

"Three sisters, each mothers of young children, were killed in a hor-rific car crash in Hyde Park last Friday . . . It's unclear what exactly caused the crash, but police said that alcohol may have been a factor."[3]

"A teenager killed when a car traveling at 115 mph in a 30 mph zone smashed into the side of a building had been given the all clear from cancer just a month before. An inquest in Bradford, West Yorkshire, heard cancer survivor Jade Best, 19, was killed with two friends when the high-powered car driven by Adam Ruthven, 27, lost control and skid-ded sideways into a hairdressing salon . . . Just days before the accident in Bradford, Miss Best—who was a backseat passenger in the car—had celebrated her 19th birthday."[4]

"Three women and a 10-year-old girl were killed in a car crash in C. Westmeath this morning."[5] I thought that the date of the accident must be wrong, since it was listed as one day in the future. I then realized that the accident happened in Europe, and due to the difference in time zones it was listed as the next day. I'm actually finding young women who are dying tomorrow. Heartbreaking.

"Charges are pending for a motorist who crashed into a tree killing a woman and injuring himself and a four-year-old boy early Sunday in the Medical Village neighborhood on the Near West Side, police said."[6]

One of the most infamous cases of a victim, a young woman, being in the wrong place, at the wrong time, with the wrong person, was Mary Jo Kopechne. She died when she accepted a ride from Teddy Kennedy after a party at a hotel. Kennedy subsequently drove off a bridge and into a channel. He was able to break free and swim to shore. He didn't report the incident until the next morning. Mary Jo had drowned in the car. Teddy Kennedy was well-known and went on to be a US senator for forty-six years. Hardly anyone even remembers Mary Jo's name.

In just the past month, another precious eighteen-year-old young woman, a student from the University of Virginia, went missing. She was last seen walking home alone after a night of partying. The exact details of her case are not yet known. No one but her murderer will ever know exactly what happened to her during her last hours.

I subsequently learned that her remains were eventually found on an abandoned property in Albemarle County and then positively identified. A suspect has been arrested and charged for her murder and is also a suspect in the death of another female student. He was previously accused of raping students at Liberty University and Christopher Newport University in 2002 and 2003, but the cases were dropped.[7] Her parents issued a statement: "We are devastated by the loss of our beautiful daughter." Her name is Hannah Graham. Will anyone but her family and friends remember the name? Hannah Graham.

5. Remember that there is safety in numbers. Zebras, wildebeests, and yaks have all figured this out. Predators, animal or human, prefer to attack lone victims. Animal predators usually single out a victim from a herd and then attack. Intelligence officers target lone sources to build rapport and trust and to manipulate. Assassins wait until a target is alone.

A colleague of mine thought one day that it would be okay to leave alone from our base in Southern Afghanistan. When he returned, I asked him where he had been. He said that he had gone for a drive but that he had "felt perfectly safe." We had a long talk about that.

I wonder how many people feel safe right up to the point that they're dead. Terrorists, assassins, or predators actually want their intended target to feel completely safe, completely unaware, right up to that point.

A group of women attending a social event, such as party or dance at a nightclub, should consider setting up their own Danger Signals. They can agree that if one of their friends changes her hairstyle, such as putting her hair back in a ponytail, or switches her purse to her left shoulder (you are only limited by your imagination!), it means that she needs some help and a friend should come to her as soon as possible. She might not be in any threatening situation but just needs a friend to help her "escape" from a crass or rude man—maybe someone who is telling her inappropriate jokes or trying to get her to go outside with him. A friend can help her easily extricate herself from uncomfortable situations. And besides, it is fun to have secret signals!

Friends can also choose verbal signals to use if you are close enough to one another or in the same group. If one of her friends is cornered by a jerk and wants to get away, she can mention beef jerky (*jerky* for jerk) or say the name of actor Steve McQueen (from the movie *The Great Escape*), or bring up any previously-agreed-upon word or phrase (again, only limited to your imagination). Once someone has mentioned the key word or phrase, then her friend can interrupt the conversation and ask her to go to the bathroom or say that she needs to call home . . . anything. These verbal signals and cues can be just as effective and fun.

Young ladies, ask a roommate to walk home with you, especially after a late-night study session. Ask your brother to pick you up after work. Ask members of the French Club, as nerdy as they are (I was in the French Club), if you can walk home with them. Ask the young lady from your church if you can catch a ride home with her after the party. Go ahead and be a scaredy-cat. But be at least as smart as a yak.

6. Keeping your numbers safe. Stalkers look for numbers: cell phone numbers, apartment numbers, and addresses. Hackers look for passwords. Identity thieves look for social security numbers. Bad people want your numbers, even your girlfriend's numbers.

A good friend's daughter told me a story of being stalked when she was in high school. She wrote her phone number down on a friend's hand, in the presence of an older student. This male student saw the number and decided to be her stalker. He called her for weeks, at all hours of the day and night, trying to talk to her, to date her, and to track her movements.

If she had only used a system, such as this (below), then the stalker would have been stopped in his tracks, before he ever started:

Add 1 or 2 (any number, but smaller numbers are easier), to whatever number you would like to encode. The number 555-1212 would be 666-2323 (if you add 1 to each digit), or 777-3434 (if you add 2 to each digit). Then simply subtract that number from each digit when you need to dial it, or provide your social security number to an office or your bank account number when withdrawing money from the bank.

If you write the numbers down and then lose your wallet or it's stolen, a criminal who finds the slip of paper will have the wrong phone number, SSN, or bank account. Be advised, however, that your parents, who will have also read this book, might find that phone number in your purse, decode it, and identify your new boyfriend!

A good friend actually taught me a great way to commit telephone numbers to memory when we were in college. It was a system that I later used a lot in the CIA. With this system, there's no need to write numbers on paper slips or hands. It's all memorized, in your head. The tool is simple—a consonant sound is assigned to each number, as follows:

0—*se* or *ze*	5—*l*
1—*te* or *de*	6—*sh* or *ch*
2—*ne*	7—*ke* or *ge*
3—*me*	8—*fe* or *ve*
4—*r*	9—*pe* or *be*

You then add vowels between the consonants and create words, or a phrase. I found a couple of phone numbers and encoded them to something I can remember:

The number for the National Domestic Violence hotline is (800) 799-7233. Remember that it's an 800 number, toll-free (unless you can come up with something for the first 3 digits), and then encode the rest: "KeeP BuGGiN' MoM," or it could be "KeeP BaCKiN' MoM (The two *g*'s in *buggin'* only count for one number because it is only one sound.) Think of it as urging her to seek help, bugging her to get assistance, or backing her with help if she's being abused.

Sometimes your code will work perfectly; other times it will not be completely logical, but sillier phrases will often stick in your memory even longer just because they are silly. I still remember some codes from thirty years ago because they are odd. Isn't it interesting that I can remember those numbers but cannot remember what I had for breakfast.

Here are a few aides to memorize the key: *ze* is like zero, 1 point after a TD (touchdown), the next four numbers (2–5) spell NuMeRaL, *s* in *six* sounds like *ch/sh*, think seven kegs, 8 like FaVor-eight, 9 (p, b). You might come up with your own way to memorize the numbers. Once you've memorized the key, however, the rest is easy and you'll have a memory tool for life.

Try it on your own social security number (SSN) or school number. Practice. Try it now. What number is hidden in "Be SaFe"? Or "SPy SchooL (*ch* can represent a "K" sound) FoR GiRLS"? Remember: only consider consonant sounds. (Answers can be found at the end of the chapter.)

7. Do not go straight home if you think you're being followed. If you've confirmed surveillance and you know that you're being followed, then don't go straight home. Going home or to your college dorm room might just compound the problem because your pursuer then knows where you live. It might be better to drive to a public area: airport, hospital, student center, gas station, or better yet, the police station—any place where you can find help.

Try to get his license plate number. If he's following you, read it off his license plate using your rearview mirror when he approaches you at a corner or red light. Just read the plate backward in your mirror. Practice it on other cars when you're driving around town. But be aware of the road in front of you! Look at the number through your mirror when you're stopped at a light. It takes practice, but you can do it.

Learn to recognize makes and models of vehicles by their logos; for example, can you identify the following logos?

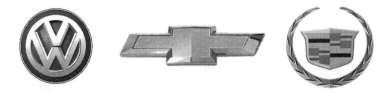

Try to obtain a detailed description of the occupants of the vehicle (the number of occupants and their sex, race, complexion, color of hair, type of clothes, and so on).

If someone is following you in a vehicle or on foot (through a shopping mall for instance), try to get a good description, including approximate height (if you're not good at judging height then compare his height to your dad or your brother), weight, hair color, facial hair, scars or tattoos, build (athletic or not), and clothing. The police have a much better chance of apprehending someone with a good description.

Again, if you're being followed in a mall or on foot, then go to mall security, a librarian, custodian, or a clerk in a store and tell them you need help. Ask them to call the police or escort you to your car. How embarrassing that might be! Not! Better safe and embarrassed than sorry.

8. Last caution: guard your drink. If you are in a nightclub or restaurant, always keep an eye on your drink. A sexual predator can slip a drug into your drink in the blink of an eye. YouTuber Joey Salads showed how quickly a man can drug a woman, merely by waiting until she leaves her drink to go to the restroom or gets distracted.[8] Don't be distracted around strangers. Don't accept drinks from strangers. Don't leave your drink alone with anyone whom you do not know. If you've left it somewhere, toss it and buy another one. The cost of a mistake with a predator—which might be rape—is much higher than the cost of a drink.

Girls, be smart and cunning. Be cunning like a fox.

1. Vary your times, routes, and donkeys!
2. Dress the part.
3. Stop and wait before you get too close to something suspicious.
4. Don't be at the WPWTWP.
5. Remember that there is safety in numbers.
6. Keep your numbers safe.
7. Do not go straight home if you think you're being followed.
8. Guard your drink.

(Answers: 908, 09075847450, Volkswagen, Chevrolet, Cadillac)

NOTES

1. Gwen Moore, "The Campus SaVE Act: A Critical Step to Ending Violence Against Women," August 16, 2012, gwenmoore.house.gov.

2. Dailymail.co.uk, "Young Woman, 21, killed in car crash that left her sister, 18, in a coma five days before her high school graduation," March 23, 2014.

3. Losangeles.cbslocal.com, "3 Sisters Killed in Car Crash Leaving Behind 5 Children," February 8, 2012.

4. Telegraph.co.uk, "Teen killed in car crash was given all-clear from cancer one month earlier," February 23, 2014.

5. Independent.ie, "Three women and a 10-year-old girl killed in horrific car crash," June 29, 2014.

6. Chicago.cbslocal.com, "Woman Dies After Car Accident," December 26, 2010.

7. Foxnews.com, "Jesse Matthew charged in Hannah Graham's murder; DA will not pursue death penalty," February 10, 2015.

8. Joey Salads, "Roofied Drink (Social Experiment)," June 1, 2015, https://www.youtube.com/watch?v=GTd1647CTFs.

16

Break the Habit

"Lord grant me chastity . . . but not yet."[1]

—St. Augustine

I do not really hate young men. They are not our enemies. They are, after all, our future sons-in-law, fathers, and grandfathers. Our daughters will someday fall in love with a young man and marry him, and he will then sit at the bedside of a daughter at her bedtime, comforting, consoling, and cherishing another precious generation.

Young men are our future.

Like Joe, I can see that they are pursuing our daughters, and I resent them for that. But unlike Joe, I'm able to see that our young men are also being pursued, and I pity them for their predicament. Many are much more the prey than the predator. They're becoming casualties of a spiritual, cultural, and economic war.

When I belonged to the CIA (maybe I still do!), I used to marvel that everyday citizens were not aware of the war being waged across the globe, even during so-called peacetime. Battles between spies—dangerous skirmishes of the espionage war—continued daily. There was spy versus spy, covert officer versus terrorist, and country versus country, whether there were bullets flying or not.

There are also similarly inconspicuous (sometimes not so) cultural wars being waged, where young men are targeted as much, maybe more, than our young women. And the same weapons of espionage are being used against them: misinformation, propaganda, disguise, misdirection, deceit, and even brainwashing.

It's a confusing war. One generation ago, our young men were taught to respect women, protect them, and cherish them. I am not that old (contrary to what my children think), but I was taught by parents, school teachers, and church leaders, to walk next to the curb when escorting a young lady down a sidewalk, to offer an elderly lady my chair, and to not just open a car door for a lady but also to avert my eyes—to look away— while she enters or exits a vehicle in order to allow her privacy as she draws her legs inside and arranges her dress. My, how the world has changed.

And it must be a confusing world to grow up in. Young women are now taught that they should not only be immodest but glory in it, even "shout it from the rooftops." Surgical procedures draw attention. Immodest clothes worn over enhanced figures draw more attention. Tight-fitting outfits with strategically placed lettering draw maximum attention. They might as well wear an outfit with arrows directing men to "look here."

There's not much averting of eyes happening in our society anymore.

It is not just confusing for the young men. It is a veritable visual minefield out there for the older guys. It's difficult to speak with women in a gym, given what most are wearing. Low-cut here, high-cut there, tight everywhere. The spandex seems to scream, "Hey, look down here!" while our old-fashioned decency shouts back, "Whoa, cowboy, avert your eyes!"

And how can young men not look? They want to be good, like St. Augustine, but they're constantly bombarded by messages that tell them women are objects to satisfy their desires, creatures to be exploited rather than cherished. They're taught that women are playmates—not their friends with whom they shared the sandbox of their youth but playmates of another kind.

And it's not just sex. Propaganda of all kinds permeates the war zone. Messages, visible and subliminal, constantly shower our society, persuading young men that violence is cool, violence is power, violence is the solution to most conflicts, and violence is the means and the end. Violent video games bring death to zombies, vampires, monsters, enemies, and terrorists.

There's so much violence in our society that terrorists must wonder how they can continue to terrorize. Westerners have seen it all in the violent video games, movies, and TV programs. Terrorist chants of "Death to America, death to everyone!" are now met with yawns.

The agents of influence—in spy terms—of this war are many: music videos, Internet pornography, movies, books, billboards, even school textbooks, and they all beat the same drum: sex is love, violence is power, sex is love, violence is power . . .

And young men—our future fathers—are fed their daily doses and are slowly but surely brainwashed. Sadly, they're also slowly conditioned to abuse our daughters.

Far from being afraid of our young men, I am afraid for them.

I am afraid for them because they're under siege. Try to find a movie that doesn't show violent images in the form of aliens, ax murderers, or a constantly rotating selection of various scenes of death and ways to die. Books and screenplays feed the movie industry with endless plots based on how victims meet their deaths, scenes that are then fed to our young, vulnerable men.

And between the scenes of death are other images based on sex: rape, prostitutes, bondage, cheating spouses, and soft or hard pornography. All of these are found in movies, on the Internet, music videos, or cable television.

When I was a young boy, I watched the following TV programs that came out that year, 1964, fifty years ago:

Bewitched—"A witch married to an ordinary man can't resist using her magic powers to solve the problems her family faces."[2] No sex or violence.

Gilligan's Island—"Seven men and women are stranded on an uncharted island following a torrential storm."[3] No sex (except for Ginger's revealing dress!) or violence.

The Addams Family—"The misadventures of a blissfully macabre but extremely loving family."[4] No sex or violence.

Flipper—Stories center on Ranger Porter Ricks, his two sons, Sandy and Bud, and their pet dolphin, Flipper. No sex or violence.

The Munsters—"A family of friendly monsters have misadventures, never quite realizing why people react to them so strangely."[5] No sex or violence.

Jonny Quest—"The Quest family and their bodyguard investigate strange phenomena and battle villains around the world."[7] No sex, very little violence.

Daniel Boone—"Frontier hero Daniel Boone conducts surveys and expeditions around Boonesborough . . . before and during the Revolutionary War."[8] No sex, little or no violence.

All the above programs were new must-see TV programs that began in 1964, none of which revolved around violence or sex.

The new movies of 1964 were even more yawn-inducing, according to today's standards, and included the following:

Mary Poppins . . . no sex or violence.
My Fair Lady . . . no sex or violence.
and the most violent—James Bond in *Goldfinger*.

A short fifty years later, in 2014, our movies are mostly forgettable but push the same two themes: sex and violence.

The Other Woman
Sex Tape
Jersey Shore Massacre
another *Expendables*.

TV shows of 2014 have sunk even further:

The Affair (The effects of an affair between a married waitress and a teacher.)
The Strain (It's about vampires. The promotional posters showed a worm emerging from a lady's eye and were withdrawn due to complaints)
Z Nation (This one is about zombies.)
Stalker (Surprise—it's about stalkers.)
Murder in the First (You guessed it—it's about murder.)
How to Get Away With Murder (Yes, it's about murder.)

The titles of this year's movies and TV shows are rather obvious regarding the content. It might not be long before Hollywood skips any pretense and just names the programs "More Sex and Violence!"

Astoundingly, Lucille Ball was not allowed to use the word *pregnant* in *I Love Lucy*. The 2014 TV line-up includes a program called *Jane the Virgin*, a show about a young lady who is accidentally, artificially impregnated by her gynecologist with sperm belonging to a former crush and present boss. Lucy must be turning over in her grave.

How do boys and men stand a chance against the onslaught of this filth? There doesn't appear to be anywhere for them to hide.

Even Fox News, a conservative news network, has found it necessary to join the craze, or cash in on it, and offers its own edgy stories in its "Features and Faces" and "See It" sections. Take a look at the news found fit to print the same day I am writing this: an article titled "Bond

Girls Gone Bad" (all about their sexual scandal and infidelity), next to "Kim (Kardashian) goes too far with Corset?" and later, "Kardashian Thanks her Loyal Fans with Thong Selfie," or "Miley Show Banned: Too Raunchy," above another article in the Fox News magazine titled "See It: Sharknado Actress is Falling out of her Dress." What young man won't click on that?[8]

The same day, I found a piece called, "Emily: I Pose Nude for Women." I clicked and read the Blurred Lines video model explain that we just "need to get over naked women." Wow, that is irony at its finest. She poses nude, asking men to look, and then tells them to "Get over it!" Look! Don't look! Get over it! Look! Don't look! Get over it!

And later the same day, interestingly, Fox News included an article on the HBO series *Game of Thrones*, which is undoubtedly the most graphic program on TV this year. Michael Lombardo, an HBO executive, defended the sex and violence depicted on the program by saying, "It is an adult service . . . I don't think [graphic scenes] have ever been without any purpose."[9]

Well then, what is the purpose?

He continues, "We have certainly not given (the writers) an edict or a note that they need to tone down the sexual content in the show." In fact, he did not ask that they cut a scene showing the character of Jaime Lannister raping his twin sister, Cersei.

The "purpose," as Lombardo called it, is to shock. He points out the purpose of the MTV awards is not really to award prizes to the winners, but to shock, á la Miley Cyrus during last year's awards. The article lists "blood, buttocks, snakes and angry rants," not to forget Cyrus's "twerking" with Robin Thicke (whose wife has now, coincidentally, filed for divorce) as elements of past performances. The article quotes Amy Doyle, executive producer of the live telecast ceremony, who says that Beyoncé, who is slated for this year's show—more aptly called *exhibition*—"will be doing something that no other artist has ever tried to do before."[10] Wow, stay tuned!

Siege: "the act or process of surrounding and attacking a fortified place in such a way as to isolate it from help and supplies, for the purpose of lessening the resistance of the defenders and thereby making capture possible."[11]

That's an accurate definition and description of what's happening to our men. These good young men are certainly surrounded by Hollywood,

MTV, Internet, radio, sexting, and Facebook friends. They're surrounded, and resistance is lessening simply by clicking.

Good men are clicking on the images and destroying their lives. College students are dropping out of college because of pornography. Married men are losing their marriages, their careers, and their lives all because they click on an image. A leader of a youth congregation in my church was asked how many young men he interviews have had trouble, or addiction, with pornography. He did not hesitate as he answered, "Nine out of ten." Sadly, one young man who first claimed that he did not have a problem with pornography later admitted to making it . . . producing pornographic videos.

Think about it: these images being forced upon our young men are merely mirages. Wikipedia notes that the word *mirage* comes from the French *mirage*, from the Latin *mirari*, meaning "to look at, to wonder at." It continues, "A mirage is a real optical phenomenon. . . . What the image appears to represent, however, is determined by the interpretive faculties of the human mind . . . images on land are very easily mistaken for reflections from a small body of water."[12] The image is an illusion.

Mirages are fascinating. I grew up in the desert where mirages are quite common. I remember walking across hot sand when hunting lizards, feeling thirsty and exhausted, and seeing mirages shimmering in the distance—always in the distance. They looked exactly like cool pools of water, and we often dreamed of running to them and jumping in, we were so thirsty. We even tried a few times.

But as you walk toward a mirage, it will recede further and further into the distance. You can never reach one. What appears to be a cool, refreshing lake will simply disappear the more you pursue it, whether you are walking or even running, depending upon the "interpretive faculties" of your mind.

Pornography is nothing but a mirage. It will draw in a thirsty traveler with the same promise of refreshment, or satisfaction, only to leave him more thirsty, exhausted, empty, and ashamed than he already was. In fact, studies have concluded that an addiction to pornography can leave a man addicted but sexually impotent, destroying the very thing that he is looking for.[13] He's left with an illusion—a mirage—which never quenches his thirst but actually worsens his condition the more he chases it. He becomes addicted to the images and to the pleasure-inducing drugs of his own mind.

As young boys, we learned to not chase mirages in the desert. If we could only learn to stop chasing other mirages in life as adults.

It's fascinating that some men who refrain from watching pornography will readily watch violence. My oldest son joined the Boy Scouts when he was twelve. He was always anxious to attend, especially when the group

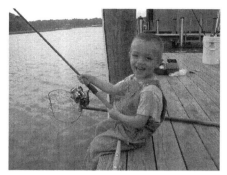

Let's protect our sons too! Here is our youngest, fishing in Virginia.

went to the scoutmaster's home to work on various projects or "bake cookies." One evening I decided to go over to the house and see how good the cookies really were. It turned out that the wife was indeed in the kitchen baking cookies, but the Boy Scout leaders and boys were divided into three groups in three different rooms, on three different TVs that were all linked together, playing a very violent video game, especially for twelve-year-olds.

When I expressed my concerns that it was inappropriate for the boys to be watching and playing violent video games, the Scoutmaster acted a little surprised. I don't think that he would've had them over to watch porn, but violence seemed acceptable.

Do we not know that we have to protect our young men, that they need our protection, and that they are precious too? If for no other reason, we need to protect them to protect our daughters.

Our daughters are also under siege. Studies have shown that young ladies are increasingly falling victim to the same addictions as men: pornography and violent video games. Maybe it's a result of hanging out with young men at homes, watching the same programs, and listening to the same music. But we can't put all the blame on our men. For whatever the reason, women are becoming hooked on the same addictions. They're not somehow immune while watching sex and violence. They either enjoy watching a zombie eat a man's face, or sit and scream, tolerating it while seated next to a young man who enjoys it.

Some young men and women will justify watching pornography by saying that it doesn't hurt anyone. Nothing could be further from the truth. It's damaging the actors and others who produce the video. It's also hurting the person watching it. Sadly, it's even hurting our children.

Timothy Ballard runs Operation Underground Railroad, which special-
izes in rescuing children trapped in slavery, and he noted, "The problem
of child sex slavery is 100 percent the societal consequence of our pornographic world . . . Pornography is a drug. Adult pornography is marijuana,
and child pornography is the cocaine."[14]

Some men believe that they can hide an addiction to pornography.
That might be easier said than done. Two college-age women advised that
they can tell if a young man is addicted to pornography:

- He might display low self-esteem
- He might act depressed
- He will tell or laugh at inappropriate jokes
- He might show signs of addiction to his cell phone or other
  mobile devices

I wish that there were spiritual safety goggles that a person could slip
on during a program, like shooting glasses at a firing range, or a welding
mask for especially gruesome scenes—something that would protect the
eyes and spirit when sex or violence shows up on the screen. But there are
not. And the viewer sees it all.

And once that viewer has seen violence or pornography, it can't be
unseen. That filth travels through once-innocent eyes, along optic nerves,
to the brain, to memory, where it stays recorded . . . for a very long time.
And it becomes part of that young man or young woman—the blood
flowing, the heads rolling, the zombies eating brains. . . . That's how
the brain works. It's a super-computer that takes it all in, commits it to
memory, and backs it up to make sure the information isn't lost. The pornography and violence are the viewer's to keep.

A young woman needs to decide what she wants to keep—or download—to her brain. If she doesn't want to have those kind of brain
"viruses," then she should get up off the couch and tell her friends that she
doesn't want to have images of brain-eating zombies or scenes of bondage
and masochism polluting her brain. She can suggest, bravely, that they
watch *Mary Poppins* or a good spy movie (*Goldfinger!*) to brush up on her
spy skills. And maybe her friends are waiting for someone else to be brave
enough to say enough is enough.

And if the boys do not agree, then find some other company.

> 'Twas an evening in November, as I very well remember,
> I was strolling down the street in drunken pride,

But my knees were all a-flutter,
And I landed in the gutter
And a pig came up and lay down by my side.
Yes, I lay there in the gutter
Thinking thoughts I could not utter
When a lady passing by did softly say,
"You can tell a man who boozes
By the company he chooses"
And the pig got up and slowly walked away.

—The Pig, by anonymous

A young woman or man can choose to be in good company. They can protect themselves from the alarming amount of violence and pornography that permeate our society. They can avoid others who enjoy violence and pornography. They can protect their eyes, souls, and innocence.

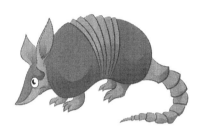

A favorite animal of mine, the armadillo of Texas, will roll up in a ball when threatened. You can do as they do, and close your eyes and ears to bad influences.

NOTES

1. St. Augustine of Hippo, Wikipedia.org.

2. "Bewitched," http://www.imdb.com/title/tt0057733/.

3. "Gilligan's Island," http://www.imdb.com/title/tt0057751/?ref_=fn_al_tt_1.

4. "The Addams Family," http://www.imdb.com/title/tt0057729/?ref_=fn_al_tt_2.

5. "The Munsters," http://www.imdb.com/title/tt0057773/?ref_=fn_al_tt_1.

6. "Jonny Quest," http://www.imdb.com/title/tt0057730/?ref_=fn_al_tt_1.

7. "Daniel Boone," http://www.imdb.com/title/tt0057742/?ref_=fn_al_tt_1.

8. Foxnews.com, August 22, 2014.

9. Leo Barraclough, "HBO Exec Defends Scenes of Sex and Violence in 'Game of Thrones,'" August 22, 2014, http://variety.com/2014/tv/global/hbo-exec-defends-scenes-of-sex-and-violence-in-game-of-thrones-1201288261/.

10. Sinha-Roy, Piya, Reuters, "So you think you can shock? Prizes take backseat at MTV awards," August 22, 2014.

11. s.v. "siege," freedictionary.com.

12. Wikipedia.com, "Mirage," accessed September 2, 2015.

13. Elizabeth Waterman, "Are You Watching Too Much Porn?" August 21, 2013, http://www.mensjournal.com/health-fitness/health/are-you-watching-too-much-porn-20130821.

14. Jamie Armstrong, "Hope Among Shadows," *LDS Living*, March/April 2015.

17
Fight

"For me there are only two kinds of women:
goddesses and doormats."[1]

—Pablo Picasso

I never did care for Picasso as a painter, and after reading about his treatment of women, I find that I dislike him even more as a person and a man. He reportedly drove at least two of his mistresses to mental illness and two others to suicide. What a Gweebi.

I quote him above for one purpose: to purposely anger the women who will read this book. I want a young woman to know that there are many Picassos in the world—plenty of them with plenty of money—who consider women their personal playthings, merely objects for their desire and nothing more. They consider women "doormats" and will wipe their feet and then move on. Women should be disgusted at that kind of attitude.

Actually, I want young women to get fighting mad at such an attitude. And be ready to fight, if necessary. If a young woman has walked across campus with her head high and shoulders straight, has continuously varied her routes and times, was as alert as a gazelle and menacing as a porcupine and watched like a hawk, did not exhibit any vulnerabilities, does not date predators or Picassos, and has done about everything a young lady can do to protect herself, she might still be a target and may need to fight.

She might be a target of opportunity, which is someone a predator spots by chance and decides to act then and there without any target selection, planning, surveilling, or anything. He might just see her walking across campus or at the gym, think she's an object to satisfy him, and decide to target her right then and there.

But since the woman he is targeting has spy skills, she is already in condition Yellow, and when those alarm bells go off in her head, she quickly moves to Orange and, if necessary, Red. And when she arrives at condition Red, she also arrives at that decision she has to make: to escape or to fight.

I put escape first because that should be our first choice, even for a 230-pound man who knows how to handle himself. I am afraid that our culture has convinced some young women that they can take martial arts or self-defense classes and can manage a jumping spin-kick to a much larger assailant's head, sending him flying across the warehouse and knocking him out. After all, Xena the Princess Warrior, Wonder Woman, Katniss, and the Black Widow of the Avengers do it all the time. And let's not forget that tough lady pilot from Avatar.

I suppose it might be empowering for young ladies to watch. But one unintended, unfortunate consequence of all these scenes of women knocking out men with one punch could very well be the message it sends: women are knocking out men, so men can also knock out women. Predators might feel that women are fair game.

It certainly seems like men are getting that message. CNN's Carol Costello, herself a victim of brutality toward women, penned an article in which she blasted the NFL's decision to hand down a wrist-slap to Ray Rice for knocking his then-girlfriend unconscious and dragging her from a casino elevator. He was given a two-game suspension. She compared it to the sixteen-game suspension given to another player for testing positive for marijuana.

Costello expected her friends to rally around her when assaulted by her boyfriend. Instead, most responded with "He's such a nice guy. You must have made him really mad."[2]

The constant message in movies is that not only is violence acceptable, but violence from women, with women, and against women seems to be acceptable as well—especially if she somehow did something to bring it upon herself.

Costello gave a few other statistics: one in four women will experience domestic violence during her lifetime. One-third of female homicide victims are killed by their current or former partner. Boys who witness domestic abuse are twice as likely to abuse their own partners and children when they become adults. She recounted her own experience of being thrown against a wall by a former boyfriend and knocked unconscious.

And she admitted, "I always thought I was a physically strong woman, but I could not defend myself against a man who outweighed me by 70 pounds."

At the risk of sounding sexist, a girl is just not physically capable of beating a boy in a fair fight, and a grown woman can't beat up a grown man in a fair fight. That is why Ronda Rousey, the Mixed Martial Arts (MMA) women's champion, will never fight a MMA men's champion in any weight category.

A woman should not take the decision to fight lightly. A woman should not allow herself to be drawn into bar fights with men. Or on a subway. Today, as I write this, I watched a video of a young woman yelling at and striking a much larger male, in a subway. He eventually could not take it any longer, punched her in the face, and knocked her unconscious.

A woman shouldn't punch a man for spilling a drink on her at a baseball game. She shouldn't get out of her car and yell at another driver for cutting her off (neither should a man). She shouldn't try and pull an MMA move against a stranger, someone who has probably not been taught by his daddy to never hit a woman. Unfortunately, the young thug may have actually watched his daddy beat his mother every Friday night.

So a lady who finds herself in a condition Red scenario should first try to escape: to walk away, to run, to scream and yell, to resist being pulled into a car, or to struggle to exit the car. My niece (the college track star) is strong, granted, but her first instinct should be to use her God-given legs and sprint like a "bat out of hell," as my football coach used to say.

And do not worry. No one—neither Katniss, nor the lady Avatar pilot, nor your friends—will look down on a woman for running away. And despite her embarrassment, thinking that she's only imagining the danger and shouldn't run or that she's feeling like she backed down from a bully, she won't find herself in a dirty van trying to fight off a rapist or tied up in a basement or dead in a ravine. She'll be alive and well, and she'll wake up the next morning at home with her family. And she'll feel good about being alive.

But after I've said all that, if she tried to run away from an attacker and he has her cornered in a back room, and she told him that she doesn't want to go out with him, that she doesn't want to be his girlfriend, that she wants him to leave her alone, or that she wants to leave, and he still persists, then she must fight. At this point, even if he does outweigh her by seventy pounds, she fights and screams and fights and screams some more.

And she doesn't fight fairly. She fights dirty. And she shows him that she's no doormat. She might not even be able to beat him, but she can hurt him enough to then escape.

- "Two Girls Fight Off Assailants in Separate Incidents": in one incident, "The man asked if he could pet her dog. . . . When the girl said no, he dragged her into an alley, ordering her to 'shut up' as he squeezed her neck. 'She let loose a blow like a donkey kick' hitting him in the groin, and her dog bit the man on the foot." In the second incident, within hours of the first, a man asked for directions from a teen who was waiting for the bus. Unfortunately, she accepted a ride from the assailant, who immediately pulled a knife and tied her up. "She was able to untie her hands, pick up the knife from the truck floorboard, and stab the driver in the left shoulder or rib cage, police said."[3]

- "A 21-year-old girl told sheriff's deputies she had battled with an assailant for nearly an hour . . . the girl said she had been introduced to the man at a south side tavern, where she had gone with friends to dance. He joined the party, and when the group decided to go to another tavern, she rode in his automobile. Instead of taking her to the agreed place . . . he made advances to her. When she resisted, he pulled her out of the machine, she said. As he threatened to strike her with a crank handle an automobile containing two couples drove up. The man then dropped the crank handle and drove away."[4]

- From the same day, same newspaper . . . "The other girl, 20, told police that she met a man in a bowling alley Sunday night. He promised to take her home in his car. Instead he drove to N. 60th and W. Hampton Rd., and attempted to attack her, she said. She succeeded in breaking away and ran down the road. He followed in his car, seized her and again attempted to assault her, she said. She again broke away, and after reaching home, notified police."[5]

Assaults on women have been going on since well before drivers needed a crank handle (a handle inserted into the engine) to start the vehicle. How many women were assaulted when men drove up on a chariot and asked her if she needed a ride to the pyramids? It has been happening since the beginning of time.

- "The two California teenage girls who were abducted Thursday tried to kill their kidnapper by stabbing him and hitting him on the head with a whiskey bottle, one of the teens said yesterday . . . 'We got this plan we were going to try to kill him,' 17-year-old Jacqueline Marris, tearfully told KABC-TV . . . 'we got enough courage . . . we both kicked him out and I threw the knife at him' . . . Deputies eventually shot and killed Ratliff.[6] A County Sheriff noted that Ratliff was 'hunting for a place to kill 'em and bury 'em.'"[7]

These girls "got enough courage" and kicked and fought for their lives. That is the way to fight: with any weapon you can find, with every ounce of your strength, for as long as it takes to escape with your life. It's important to decide that is how you will react long before it happens. Make the decision now.

Everyone in the country felt terribly for Elizabeth Smart. I know that every situation is different, but who knows what would've happened if she had screamed and fought and kicked and scratched and gouged Brian Mitchell's eyes. Or if her sister had screamed. They were young and extremely frightened; fear can paralyze a victim. But what if she had fought or screamed at the top of her lungs?

Scientists discovered that fear can release a "cocktail" of chemicals in the bloodstream that actually paralyzes a victim, at least for a short time. That is probably what happened to Elizabeth. It must have been the most terrifying thing that can happen to a young lady.

A lion's roar can freeze a gazelle for a split-second, just enough time for the lion to catch and kill his prey. American Indians reportedly screamed during attacks. So did Maori warriors. The rebel yell was a battle cry used by Confederate soldiers to scare the Yankees.

So, women, do everything in your power to overcome that fear—that chemical cocktail dump—during that split-second after an attack. Tell yourself quickly that you must not get in the car, must not go with him, must not set foot on his X or that you need to quickly get off his X if you are already standing on it.

And quickly turn that fear into anger and a savage desire to survive.

You want to go home again and be with your family. So fight for yourself, for them, and for your life. Get fighting mad. Girls, fight like a tiger.

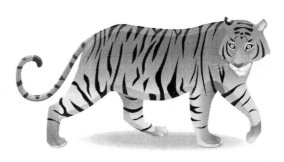

NOTES

1. Annabel Venning, "How Picasso who called all women goddesses or doormats drove his lovers to despair and even suicide with his cruelty and betrayal," Dailymail.co.uk, March 7, 2014.

2. Carol Costello, "Rice 'punishment': What is NFL thinking?" Cnn.com, July 26, 2014.

3. Kieran Nicholson and Tom McGhee, "Two girls fight off assailants in separate incidents," Denverpost.com, June 12, 2014, http://www.denverpost.com/news/ci_25949466/edgewater-cops-teen-girl-stabs-kidnapper-escapes-ordeal.

4. *Milwaukee Journal*, September 27, 1937

5. *Milwaukee Journal*, September 27, 1937

6. David K. Li, "Kidnap girls tried to kill fiend," August 3, 2002, http://nypost.com/2002/08/03/kidnap-girls-tried-to-kill-fiend/.

7. CNN.com, "Sheriff: Rescued girls were minutes from death," August 2, 2002, http://www.cnn.com/2002/US/08/01/teen.abduction/.

18

Vulnerability of Feeling Invulnerable

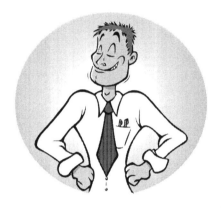

I wonder if all those movies of kick-butt women and years of empowerment has not left many ladies with the distinct impression that they have plenty of power to deal with bad men. They might even feel an acute sense of confidence or overconfidence. Many might start to believe that they are physical or spiritual superheroes: they can walk where they want to walk, talk to whomever they want to talk, and are just plain invincible.

This feeling of invulnerability, as far as emotions go, might be more dangerous than feeling vulnerable. A feeling of invulnerability might lead someone to think that she is safe, just like in the movie *GoldenEye* when the villain, Boris Grishenko yells near the end of the movie, "Yes, I am invincible!" right before he's sprayed with liquid nitrogen and is frozen solid. Famous last words.

I find it interesting to hear witnesses and victims on TV reports recount that they "felt safe" (like my colleague in Afghanistan) right up to the instant before an attack or a shooting. The victim notes that the attacker seemed like such a nice neighbor, and they're all shocked to find bodies buried in his backyard. But seriously, feeling completely safe is really an unsafe feeling. People who walk around in condition White usually feel safe. "Ignorance is bliss," after all. A young lady in condition White feels completely safe and blissful, right up to the point a stalker appears in her window or an older man tries to sexually assault her after she breaks up with a boyfriend.

And this feeling of invulnerability is often accompanied by an attitude of "It could never happen to me," which is just as dangerous.

I have told my wife many times before trips that I will be careful because I have an attitude that it *could* happen to me. Therefore, I am *less vulnerable* because I know that *I am vulnerable.*

I once traveled to Africa with a group of men. During our stay, one of them began talking about hiring prostitutes at the end of the trip to celebrate the completion of our mission. He was relentless and seemed intent on wearing the rest of our team down, wanting us all as accomplices, of course. When that day arrived, we agreed to accompany him to a local nightclub for drinks. Knowing what he planned to do, however, I let everyone know that I would drive a separate vehicle so that I could return to our residence when I wanted and by myself.

As soon as I walked into the bar, four women hurried toward us and sat at our table. I immediately told the woman who sat down next to me, politely, that I was there for a short time, and that I would be going home, alone. She did not believe me and sat next to me while I had my soda. After a while, I excused myself and drove home alone.

About an hour later, my three colleagues drove up to our residence in their vehicle with their three prostitutes. At the beginning of that trip, they must have all felt safe, and each of them, except the ringleader, must have also believed "it could never happen" to him, that he would not betray his wife, that he would never bring a prostitute to a CIA safe-house, nor bring who-knows-what diseases home. Each might have had that same thought at the bar when having drinks when a woman sat next to him. As the night wore on and the alcohol flowed, they probably felt even more and more safe.

Each of them was wrong. It could happen, and it did.

Fifteen years later, I ran into one of the three on another assignment overseas in a war zone. His initial look of surprise and happiness to see me was quickly replaced by a drop in his demeanor. I could tell that he still felt bad about that night, years earlier, just by the look in his eye. And I felt bad too. I felt sorry that I hadn't tried to persuade him to return to the safe house with me.

Another colleague was serving in an Eastern European country in the early 1990s. The head of the government's presidential security invited him out for drinks. He agreed, and as the night wore on and the alcohol flowed, the two decided to leave with their two prostitutes. He might have even felt safe when they left the restaurant—right up to the point that an armed militiaman at a road block lifted his AK-47 as their vehicle passed by and fired off three rounds. He must have felt safe, right before one of the bullets hit him in the back of his head.

I do not know what he was thinking, but it was probably "it could never happen to me," or he would not have gone with them and would have been home with his wife.

Did Prince Charles ever believe that he could end up cheating on his wife, Princess Diana, or that she would die in a horrific automobile accident in a French tunnel? He's the prince, of course, and that could never happen to a prince—at least not in the movies. Did she, the princess, believe that it could ever happen to her?

It's okay for a person to feel a little unsafe—to believe that it could happen. I know that I can't allow myself to be in inappropriate or risky situations with other women, to have lunch with another woman, or to drive somewhere with another woman. I also know that I shouldn't play on the freeway. Or poke a tiger with a stick. Or be in a room alone with chocolate. I don't feel safe around chocolate. I have a hard time resisting chocolate, and I often tell my children to not give me another piece, no matter how much I plead or beg for it. I know that I can be vulnerable.

It's okay for a young woman to feel a little unsafe and powerless, especially when she's around a man she doesn't know well. It's even okay for an empowered young woman to feel a little cautious when dating a young man that she does know fairly well but is still vetting. Feeling a little unsafe is safe. Feeling a little powerless can be empowering.

19

Intervention

Blaine was a funny classmate of ours at Kearns High School. How funny was he, you might ask? He was so funny that each day during lunchtime, he would perform for other students, his classmates, two full rows of boys seated along the hallway heaters. He was so funny that he would regularly imitate any animal of our choosing—a cow, pig, monkey, or dog—whatever animal we suggested. And we boys would all laugh and cheer him on. He was the life of the party.

Blaine would do it for attention and, more likely, so we would be his friends. You see, Blaine had no real friends, so he needed us desperately. And he was willing to do desperate things to have friends. He was willing to make a fool of himself, crawling on all fours down the hall, snorting or mooing or barking. And we were willing to manipulate him by exploiting his vulnerability.

You see, Blaine was mentally disabled. And sadly, this spectacle happened over and over, during many lunches. It went on day after day, week after week. And nobody stopped it. It went on and on until a teacher found him dead one afternoon, his lifeless body lying at the bottom of the Kearns High School swimming pool.

I have never forgotten being there while he barked and mooed, day after day, and not doing anything about it. I have not forgotten him, or what we did to him, for the past forty years. I remember how I knew that it was wrong, and how I did nothing to stop it.

It would've taken courage to stop it. I would've had to choose sides— to stand against my friends and side with the "retard," as he was called. It would've been difficult to go against all those guys. But I could've done it. I should've stood up for him.

A young woman must be brave to rescue someone with a vulnerability. But she must first be observant. The same observation skills that a young lady can use to protect herself can also be used to protect her friends, other young women, or young men. An alert young woman who can spot and avoid a "hustler" can also spot a friend being hustled or a friend that's vulnerable to a hustle.

It's not always that easy to notice someone who is vulnerable or some-one who needs help. Some people suffer in silence—remaining members of that "secret society of abuse." They keep their agony, pain, or vulner-abilities hidden.

But the alert young woman with spy skills can notice that a young lady in her circle of friends is increasingly quiet, despondent, depressed, or isolated. She might notice that the young lady is withdrawing from social contact. She might notice a change in personality or comments like, "I don't want to live anymore." A friend needs to react to any of these signs by talking to the young lady or to a parent or professional. If the signs are serious enough, it might indicate that the young lady is considering hurting herself.

There are often signs, maybe subtle ones, that an observant young lady will notice. Her friend might be dressing differently; she might be acting more promiscuously. She might hurt herself. This vulnerable young lady might begin drinking, using drugs, doing anything to fit in, to go along with the crowd, or to make herself more attractive to young men, usually the wrong kind of young men.

An observant woman will see these changes, these signs, or "red flags," and will step in to help. A true friend, especially a woman with enhanced *paratiritikotita* (remember that word?), will notice the pain another woman is feeling and then take immediate steps to alleviate it.

Once a girl has been observant and sees a friend in trouble, the next step is courage. She needs to be brave in the face of potential ridicule. It's difficult to stand against a crowd to protect someone who is vulnerable. It's hard to go up to the captain of the football team, who is probably surrounded by his teammates, or the head cheerleader and her "posse," and tell them to leave someone alone. It can be difficult to approach a vulnerable young woman at a party and tell her, "Hey, I think you've had enough," or, "Can you come to the bathroom with me? I need to talk to you," or whisper in her ear, "Don't go with him. I can give you a ride home."

If she is afraid to intervene, she can enlist others to help her. She should let others know that someone is in trouble and needs help, immediately: tell other friends at the party, the lifeguard at the pool, a teacher on the class trip, or the police. The potential victim should not be left alone, nor should a rescuer! Not only is there safety in numbers, there is strength in numbers.

It can be difficult to choose sides, especially when choosing between popularity and humiliation. It can be a big risk. A young woman can risk her status and could end up "demoted" from the cool club. A young rescuer might be relegated to the unpopular, geek clique from that moment on. Not a pleasant thought. But while the vulnerable girl and her rescuer will both be together in the geek clique, neither of them will be in that secret society of abuse. Now that's a nice thought.

And it's a much better thought than guilt. Take it from me. It's much better to pay attention to the voice that whispers to you that a precious young lady needs help, than hear another voice repeat for forty years, "You could have helped."

I've tried to redeem myself. I don't know that we can make up for past sins. We can only try to not make the same mistakes.

One morning my son and I were hurrying the couple of blocks from our home, in a European city, to his bus stop, which was next to a subway stop. By some miracle, as parents with children can all relate to, we made it to the stop that day with time to spare.

I began giving a last-minute quiz to my son: "Do you have your lunch? Do you have your homework? Did you brush your teeth?" As I was talking and he was rolling his eyes, I spotted the daughter of a colleague, Jeanne, a pretty young girl of thirteen or fourteen, speaking to a man near some benches in a small park next us. As I watched, I wondered why she wasn't moving toward the bus, and then realized that she was trying to walk around him—but he kept blocking her path. I told my son to stay where he was and walked the few steps over to Jeanne.

I first asked her how she was and she replied, nervously, that she was fine. I then asked the man, "Who are you?"

He replied in a belligerent tone and with a defiant look, "Nobody."

I was surprised at first by his response, but then quickly realized that he was someone harassing her, so I told him that she had to leave right then to board the school bus, which had just arrived. He replied, in a now angry tone, that he was not finished speaking with her.

I can still remember trying to reason with him, while going down a mental checklist, giving him a sufficient number of chances before fighting:

"Listen, Mr. Nobody, she is a student in school and is going to miss the bus."

"She is too young for you."

"Her dad is huge (and a rugby player), so don't mess with her."

Most of his responses consisted of "So what," "I don't care," or, "Too bad."

His response to my last chance, "Oh, really? And what are you going to do about it?" was accompanied by a shove, which pretty much set things in motion. I pushed him back and he fell off the sidewalk curb and into traffic. A car zoomed by, narrowly missing him. He jumped back on the curb and came at me, fists in the air, trying to look like a boxer, and started swinging.

Back in those days, I wore my wedding ring on my right hand, partly because it fits my right ring finger better and partly from a habit developed living overseas in a country where that's the custom.

When my right fist connected with his left cheek, the ring cut him under his eye, and he began to bleed. He looked a little surprised that his insults had actually turned into a fight. Many in Europe prefer a lot more bouncing around in boxing mode, insulting each others' countries, sisters, mothers, and the Virgin Mary—in that order—before the fists fly.

But his shock didn't dissuade him from giving it another go, so he came at me again—only this time with his head slightly turned, as if trying to hide behind his own head. I'm no trained fighter, so "if it worked once it will work again" was about the extent of my strategy. I threw another right and he again caught it with the side of his head; he turned away just as I swung and my fist connected with his left ear.

This time he fell against a tree and slid down the trunk to a sitting position. I stood there, angry that I had become involved in another fight (this was my second one in six months), angry that it had occurred in front of my son and this girl, and angry that I now had to return home—with the children—and tell my wife that I had gotten into another fight on the way to work.

As I was standing there being angry, the would-be predator reached over for a plastic bag that he had dropped earlier and which I hadn't previously noticed. I instinctively stepped forward and kicked it down the sidewalk.

My friends advised me that I was smart to kick his bag since he could've had a weapon inside. To be honest, I did it out of anger. As the bag skidded across the sidewalk, fresh-baked croissants spilled out of the opening and scattered along the ground. In a less belligerent tone, the once rough, tough predator whined, "Leave my croissants alone." I told him that I would be glad to leave his croissants alone if he left the girl alone. He agreed.

I called my son later that day after he had returned home from school.

"How was your day?" I asked him.

"Fine," he replied.

"You're not upset about what happened this morning?"

"What?" he questioned.

"You know, the fight."

"Oh yeah, that."

"Well, that didn't bother you at all?"

"Nah, I knew you'd win."

When I think about this incident, I feel happy that I was observant, that I noticed a young lady who needed help, and that I was brave enough to act. I am also glad that I didn't get beat up in front of my son. But I am particularly happy that I stood up for someone in need.

And I still hope, after all these years later, that Blaine will forgive me for not protecting him.

Girls, protect your friends and anyone who needs a friend.

20

Congressional Parental Oversight

Girls often resist parental supervision, or "oversight" as they call it in the government. I get that. I don't like it either. I had to submit this book to my former employer, the CIA. Imagine that! It's annoying! Those people would not let me write about all the places I worked, like ███, ███, or ███. I am sure that Mr. ███ in the ███ department and Mrs. ███ in the ███ both believe they can still look over my shoulder, even after I have retired. That is ███. Who the ███ do those people think they are? What the ███?

All kidding aside, oversight can indeed be annoying. I was annoyed when the CIA returned my book looking a bit like the above paragraph. But once the annoyance subsided, and I really thought about it, I find that I completely agree with the process.

In fact, I signed up for this oversight years ago when I first joined the CIA. I took an oath to protect and defend our country and the Constitution, and I signed secrecy agreements, which contribute to the defense of our country and Constitution.

And, ladies, so did you. You signed up for oversight when you were born. And rather than feeling controlled, you need to feel loved. Because your parents have sworn to defend and protect you.

Girls, I understand why you resist oversight and sometimes feel controlled. Girls want to be women, especially independent women. You don't want your dad looking over your shoulder or asking when you're coming home, what you're planning to do, with whom you're going out, or where you're going. You can sometimes feel your parents do not trust you and that they are being controlling.

But, girls, you need to realize that oversight is a necessary part of life and protecting life and that everyone has oversight. Employees have oversight from their managers. Managers have oversight from the CEO. Students get it from teachers, the principal, and a superintendent. Basketball players get it from a coach, a general manager, the NBA owner, and the NBA commissioner—who has oversight from his wife!

CIA officers have lots of oversight, and many working there feel the same way: "Why do we have to tell you what we are doing, why we are doing it, and with whom we are doing it? Stop trying to control us! Don't you trust us?" (Okay, there was that one incident with prostitutes at a safe house).

The CIA is controlled by executive oversight in the form of the President's Foreign Intelligence Advisory Board (PFIAB), the Intelligence Oversight Board (IOB), the Office of Inspector General, the National Security Council, and by congressional oversight with its House Permanent Select Committee on Intelligence (HPSCI) and the Senate Select Committee on Intelligence (SSCI). There are probably more boards that I don't know about. Heck, there might be boards that no one knows about. But all those committees and boards and fancy offices want the same thing: they want to know who the CIA is targeting or working with, what we're doing, when we'll do it (and stop doing it), why we're doing it (it had better be worth it), and where we're doing it. How we're doing it is thrown in just for good measure.

As annoying as it can be, government oversight is necessary to protect the Agency and the country. The government is also trying to keep the CIA out of the headlines and CIA officers out of jail. They also want to prevent any diplomatic incidents, scandals, or wars.

Oversight lets the CIA know that we're being watched, that we're accountable, and that we can't act recklessly. I don't know that it works all of the time, but I do know that some of my supervisors grew very agitated, asked us lots of questions, and wore their best suits when called to Capitol Hill to testify in front of the US Congress on some sensitive matter. It can be an uncomfortable experience. And they probably try to avoid it by not acting recklessly.

A young lady should not feel that she is any less important than the CIA, especially now that she has secret spy skills. She is important enough to be watched and monitored as well, albeit on a slightly smaller scale. Young ladies are subject to similar oversight, in the form of the

Brother Oversight Board (BOB), Board of Secret Sisters (BOSS), Neighborhood Adult Group (NAG), The Senior Advisory Group, made up of grandparents (SAG), the Aunts and Uncles Watching Over Her Shoulder Committee (AUWOHSC), and the most important, the Parental Select In-Your-Face, In-Your-Business, Hovering Everywhere Council (PSIYFIYBHEC).

And these oversight committees for youth all have the same concerns, and worries: they want to keep their young ladies safe, cautious, and out of trouble. They would also like to keep the girls off the front page—at least not in the form of bad news—and especially out of the obituaries. So these boards have a need to know.

The phrase *need to know* is common in the government. It pertains to classified information and whether a person has the need to know it or not. If someone does not need the information for his job to effectively complete his work, then he should not have it. If a person needs it for a position, then he or she has the need to know and is granted access. Parents, on the other hand, have top-secret clearances regarding their children and need to know everything. Ladies, just consider your parents the NSA.

1. Who? Parents need to know who is taking their daughter on a date. Is he someone that parents can trust with the most precious person in their life? Is the young man authentic, reliable, and trustworthy? Will he get her home on time, safe and sound? Does he seem responsible and mature, or is his photo on the County Sheriff's Bookings website? (I do check it often.) Is he from a good family? It's not a foolproof question but one that can provide insights. Parents and upbringing are important.

If the young woman is smart, she'll want to introduce a young man to her parents; it can be revealing. Maybe he'll decline the invitation. If so, why? Why doesn't he come inside her home, preferring to drive up and text or honk the horn? And after he meets the parents, why does her dad love him or hate him? Why does her mom suspect something is wrong (because she sees through his disguise)? Why does her little brother jump up and down when her date arrives? (Because her date is a nice guy and treats her brother with caring, like a real person—in other words, better than she treats her brother!)

Her parents want to know the young men she dates. Actually, they're going to insist on knowing them. So since they demand to meet him, she should use it to her advantage. Vet the young man during the process, and consider it the "family ops test." Watch him to see how he acts, how he interacts, and how he treats people. See him.

2. What? Parents need to know what she's going to do that particular Friday night. They need to know if she's planning to go to the theater just down the street from her home or if she's going to drive up the canyon road with friends. They need to know that she had intended to see the movie but then changed her mind to go to a mountain cabin, where there's no cell phone coverage and no way for her to reach her parents in case of trouble. They need to know if she was invited to a party at Joe Shmoe's house—the same Joe Shmoe whose father was arrested last month for cooking methamphetamine in his basement.

Parents need to know if she's going bungie jumping, sky-diving, mudding, four-wheeling, snowboarding, ice-blocking, or quilting at the assisted living center.

3. When? Parents need to know when she's leaving and when she's returning. A young lady might be asking, Why the urgent need to know? Because parents need to know when to start worrying. If she tells them she's going to be home by midnight, then they won't be worrying at 9:00 p.m., 10:00 p.m., and 11:00 p.m. She can save her parents hours of worry. And when she arrives home on time, at midnight, she will save them hours more of stress, which they would have felt when she stayed out after her curfew.

Telling them when she'll be home from hiking could even save her life. Parents will know when to call for help or send help, park police, or Search and Rescue if she doesn't show up at her vehicle as planned. When is very important. Don't sweat the when. Parents, especially Samoan fathers, must know if he is taking her out TOO LATE! (See page 80.)

4. Why? This is just as important. When parents ask a young lady why she's going on a date with a particular young man or why she's going to the party out in the desert or why this or that movie, it gets to the heart of the matter. If a young lady finds herself not able to answer the why, or wondering, *Hmm, I actually don't know why I'm going on a date with that bozo*, or if her answer is, "Everyone else is going," then it might be time to rethink her decision.

5. Where? Parents need to know where the young lady is going. Where is just as important, or more so, since parents need to know where to send the park police, Search and Rescue, or Marines. Parents need to know if a young man is taking her TOO FAH!

Many people have heard of Aron Ralston, the young man who became trapped in a Utah canyon and had to cut off his own arm to survive. They even made a movie about him, called *127 Hours*. He was called a hero and an experienced outdoorsman. What most people don't consider, or remember, is that he made many mistakes and put himself in that predicament. It was actually a self-inflicted injury, which he has admitted.

Cliff Ransom of *National Geographic* magazine interviewed Rex Tanner, a ten-year Search and Rescue (SAR) veteran, who commented on Ralston's situation and mistakes:

> He could have left a note. He could have had a buddy. To me, one of the biggest problems out there is people don't tell someone that they're going to a particular location. It's really not that difficult to do, and to me, it doesn't take away from the wilderness experience. . . .
>
> What bothered me was the way the media made him [Ralston] out to be quite a hero. But they never talked about how the guy got himself into trouble because he really made some poor decisions. What's kind of irritating is that rescuers have to go out and deal with those types of situations—a lot—and most of the time they're preventable.[1]

Do tell your parents where you're going, when you'll be back home, whom you're going with, and leave a note if they're not home. Don't cause your parents unbelievable anguish, somewhat similar to what a stupid hiker can cause rescuers. As Tanner pointed out, "It's really not that difficult to do." And it will not take away from your dating experience either.

If the CIA can endure oversight, then so can you. Allow your parents to protect you from doing something stupid. Allow your parents to protect you from someone who might do something stupid to you. They trust you, but they don't trust others so much. Allow your parents to help you avoid the Mr. Wrongs out there.

Obedience in the CIA keeps its officers off the front pages. Obedience in the military keeps soldiers alive in battle. A little obedience can go a long way to keeping a young lady safe. So, girls, be like obedient soldiers.

Allow your loved ones to know the following:

1. Who you are going to date or will be at the party.
2. What you will be doing.

3. When you will be home.
4. Why you are going.
5. Where you are going.

NOTES

1. Cliff Ransom, "Did Climber Have to Cut Off Arm to Save Life?" July 24, 2003, http://news.nationalgeographic.com/news/2003/07/0724_030724_AronRalston.html.

21

A Man Is a Mango

I know that women find men as hard to understand, or decipher, as we do women. I think it must be challenging, which surely makes it hard for women to find a good man. It must be as hard to select a good man as it is to pick a good mango.

At Mango.org it suggests:

- Don't focus on color. It is not the best indicator of ripeness.
- Squeeze the mango gently. A ripe mango will give slightly.
- Use your experience with produce such as peaches or avocados, which also become softer as they ripen.
- Ripe mangos will sometimes have a fruity aroma at their stem ends.
- The red color that appears on some varieties is not an indicator of ripeness. Always judge by feel.[1]

That might be good advice for selecting a man, as well: don't focus on color (good men come in all colors), squeeze him gently—if mature, he will give slightly (to your wishes and to your concerns). Use your experience with other "fruit" (how does he act compared to others?) and judge by "feel."

Well, the last rule is not true 100 percent of the time, as we have noted. Feelings can often get in the way or get a young woman in trouble. As we discussed, it might be best to do some vetting, testing, and eliciting, and then throw in some feelings later.

It might seem curious to compare a man to a mango. But there are plenty of similarities, such as softening when ripe. I hope that I am becoming softer—more caring, considerate, and compassionate—as I ripen. All men take a while to ripen, like a good mango.

TAHITI TIME

I have a radio-controlled—or atomic—clock on my bedroom wall. A radio-controlled clock is supposed to be always correct, down to the second, because it receives signals from the National Institute of Standards and Technology (NIST) Radio Station WWVB, in Fort Collins, Colorado. Doesn't that sound accurate?

Our atomic clock is correct to the second but four hours behind. I don't know why. I constantly reset it and reset it, and it stubbornly remains four hours behind.

I found this really irritating until I realized that it must show the correct time somewhere, for some country. As they say, even a broken clock is correct twice a day. So I looked it up, and lo and behold, our clock shows the correct time in Tahiti.

I try and try to reset it, but it usually returns to Tahiti time. And women try and try to reset men. But we just stay on Tahiti time. To our credit, however, we keep running!

If men had a choice, we would all live on the island of Tahiti, actually. In a man's heart, he is Tahitian. Why Tahiti?

MEN LOVE BEACH ATTIRE

- He loves to wear shorts, even in the winter.
- He love flip-flops. He can feel and see his toes down there on the floor while sitting in a boring class, especially while looking for distractions. He can sit there, with his chin resting on the edge of the desk, watching his toes wiggle, almost as if they are waving, encouraging him to "hang in there, brah'; we go to the beach after class."
- With flip-flops he doesn't have to wash any socks.
- With no socks he doesn't get in trouble with his *vahine* (woman) for leaving socks on the bed, floor, or stairs.
- He doesn't have to polish his flip-flops.
- He hates to dress up. He doesn't like to shop for dress-up clothes or wear dress-up clothes. And think about it: *dress up* actually

uses the word *dress*. But seriously, even if it were called *pants up*, he still wouldn't like it.

- He doesn't like suits, unless it's a swimsuit, which includes the word *swim*. If a woman understands a man swimming at a Tahitian beach, wearing flip-flops and shorts, she can begin to understand a man.

MEN LOVE WOMEN IN BEACH ATTIRE

I was a Mormon missionary in the Tahitian and Cook Islands from 1977–79. I was homesick when I first arrived. I had never even seen the ocean until I was eighteen on my high school senior trip, and even then it was only for a few hours. The day after arriving in Papeete, the capital, other missionaries took me to the wharf and put me on an overnight boat to Raiatea. We boarded and laid our mats made of woven pandanus leaves in rows, ready for sleeping on the wooden deck.

Before long, a Tahitian family boarded and arranged their belongings next to us, their mats also laid out on the deck. Two of the mats belonged to two attractive girls—probably daughters—who were about our age. And they sat down right next to me, wearing their attractive beach attire.

The weather in Tahiti usually ranges from warm to hot, even in the evening. So it wasn't long before the two girls began to feel hot, too hot for clothes, and they started pulling off some of their beach attire. They lay down on the mats next to me, wearing nothing but their *pareus* (lava-lava) and bras. This was a little less than beach attire and more than I had ever seen. I realized that I was definitely not in Utah anymore.

As I lay there next to the two hot women, trying to sleep, and trying with all my might to concentrate on the tarp hanging above me, I thought to myself, *Seriously? I'm supposed to lie here next to two beautiful Tahitian women in their underwear for the next two days and a night? Welcome to two years of hell.*

Ironically, the English translation of Raiatea, which was our island destination, is "faraway heaven." It's funny now, all these years later, when I realize that Tahiti is more heaven than hell, but maybe not for a missionary.

MEN LOVE TO EAT

Men love food, and Tahiti has plenty of it. If a man is hungry in the Tahitian islands—or practically anywhere in the South Pacific—he can reach up and pick a mango, banana, orange, coconut, avocado (we had them growing on trees in our backyard), guava, papaya, breadfruit, or passion fruit (what man would not like a fruit named "passion"). If he doesn't feel like reaching up, he can reach down to the ground and pick taro, arrowroot, pineapple, or a number of other things. The ground is so fertile that a man can basically plant a stick in the ground and it will grow.

And the weather on Tahiti is perfect for a man. It rains just enough that food will grow, but also enough that a man can complain to his *vahine*, "Honey, it's raining, and the ground is too wet. So I can't go plant today. Maybe tomorrow." It's also sunny enough that a man can complain to his *vahine*, "Honey, it's too hot, and the ground is too dry, so I can't go plant today. Maybe tomorrow." I am not saying that we men do not work on Tahiti time, just not when it's rainy or sunny. And especially not when our ten little buddies are yelling at us to go to the beach.

Men can even find food at the beach! The ocean is a veritable grocery store of merchandise, much of which can be eaten raw. I had my first plate of raw fish when we arrived on our boat to Taha'a, one stop before Raiatea, and didn't really care for it. But a couple of years later, I found myself fishing on a reef, catching a fish, slicing it down the sides with a knife like a Polynesian friend taught me, swishing it in the ocean water to salt the meat, and eating it right off the hook. Delicious.

I played rugby on a university team in Hawaii, an all-Polynesian team, except for me. One Saturday, a few of the players missed lunch at the cafeteria, having arrived after it had closed. Understandably, they wondered where they would eat their meal. The word for *dog* in Rarotongan translates as "barking pig," and they must have thought, *Hey, we know where to find a barking pig. The dorm mother has a barking pig!* So, understandably, they caught her dog, started a fire in a grove of trees behind the campus, and cooked it. Any man will ask, why would they not eat a barking pig?

As logical as it seems for them to eat a barking pig, however, I admit that I can't picture the woman's volleyball team catching the dorm mother's dog and eating it. They probably would have just skipped their lunch. But, to us mango-brains, that would be plain strange. Miss a meal?

My first mission companion was a Tahitian named Elder Teio. One night, he told me that his grandpa had shared the family recipe for cooking missionaries, which is how they welcomed and then "prepared" them. Elder Teio explained that the Tahitians would tie the live missionary up, seat him on a bed of hot coals, and cook until tender, or their skull split open, as he described it.

I slept with one eye open after that.

A Caucasian rugby player from an opposing team once tried to pick a fight with a much larger Polynesian on my rugby team during the after-game party. (This party is usually called the "third half," and probably has as many injuries as the first two.) This is how crazy a man can become when drinking. The Polynesian inched closer, looked at him out of his scarred, scary eyes, his ham-sized fists hanging at his side, and said, "I kill you; I eat you."

I could picture the poor player all tied up in a seated position, roasting on a fire. Fortunately, the white player became even whiter and walked away.

MEN LOVE TO FIGHT

Mango men do not shy away from fights. So rugby, often an organized fight, is a favorite sport. Many of our rugby games ended after one half—not at the end of regulation but at the beginning of strangulation.

During one game, I attempted to tackle a Polynesian player on the opposing team and our heads cracked together. My head was a little lower and struck him above the eye, splitting his eyebrow open. Thinking that I had head-butted him on purpose, he jumped up quickly off the ground, fists flying, and a fight broke out. People often joke that they were "watching a fight when a rugby game broke out."

The fight was eventually stopped after a sufficient number of punches had been thrown, and the game continued.

The next day was Sunday, and I saw him—the same young man whom I fought the day before—standing on the other side of the church chapel. He was sporting a butterfly bandage over his eye. I noticed him glance my way and then immediately start walking toward me.

My first thought was, "Uh-oh, here it goes again." I truly believed that we were going to fight in the middle of church. But as he approached, I saw a big smile spread across his face. He then threw his arms around me in a big hug and exclaimed, "Eh, brah, what a great game yes-tah-day!"

Most mango men love to fight. It must be in our genes. But ladies, once we fight, it's usually over. We let off steam, get it out of our system. That's why rugby is a great game. Men get to let off steam, lots of steam, so we don't explode like a pressure cooker.

I lived with seven men in a home while going to BYU in Provo. One day, I was talking to the landlord—a nice lady—who told me that she would never, ever, rent to women again. She explained, "Boys tend to fight and then get over it. They get it out of their system and it's done. Women, on the other hand, will keep quarreling all semester."

It is true. Women might throw looks instead of punches, but the looks don't seem to let off enough steam, and the pressure remains and simmers, maybe even grows, sometimes for a long time. Interestingly, this difference in steam release sometimes gets us in trouble with our *vahine*, because we've often already let off all our steam when she's still simmering.

When mango men aren't fighting, they're laughing. We love to laugh and to tell jokes, to have parties, to roast pigs (or barking pigs), to drink a bit, sometimes too much, and to maybe fight a bit more, and then to laugh the next day at how funny the fight was.

But ladies, regarding men and fighting, don't let your man watch too much of it. Watching too much violence will only cause him to build up too much steam with no outlet. If he's playing rugby every day and getting beat up, he might not find the venting so enjoyable and will calm down. But if he isn't getting beat up in a rugby match, then help him to not watch too much violence.

MEN LOVE LOVE

Lastl to truly understand men, a lady needs to know that he might tell many girls that he loves them. He's not a liar; it's just what he feels. Some observers might call him shallow.

Women must know that men feel love differently than a woman. Maybe it's a different definition of love. Men, especially the unripe ones, often feel love more like a magician's black powder, easily lit by a spark, and poof—suddenly gone in a flash. Call us immature, shallow, unripe— yes, yes, and yes—but men do love, just not the same as women.

I believe that it has a lot to do with a God-given drive, the sex drive, which men have in abundance. The sex drive doesn't allow men to envision consequences. This sex drive is so powerful, often consuming, that it causes men to not just ignore consequences but also to not even consider them. Pregnancy? STDs? Whatever. Usually those words don't even cross his mango mind, at least not when sex takes center stage.

A few years back, my oldest son took a beautiful young lady to our pond at our farm. The two swam for a while, and I imagine that she looked pretty good in her beach attire. After drying themselves off and preparing to return to town, she asked my son if she could drive my truck. I'm sure that he didn't think twice, seeing her in beach attire, and gave her the keys. Consequences didn't even cross his mind. Beach attire was on his mind.

A few minutes later, driving down the gravel road too fast, she lost control and rolled the truck several times, and they ended up facing the other direction in the dirt on the other side of the road. Windshield smashed, top crushed. Thank heavens that they only suffered cuts and scratches from broken glass. But my Toyota Tundra was totaled.

First, he lied when he told me that he was the driver. Then he confessed that she was driving the truck. Even that was still not the truth. His sex drive was driving my truck.

I loved that truck.

Because of this sex drive, unripe mango men will say just about anything and do anything to get what they want, which is to "drive." At that moment, the girl is the most beautiful girl in the world. In his eyes (especially if he's wearing his "beer goggles"), she is the most beautiful. He will tell her that she is the most fabulous creature to ever walk the face of the earth. That he loves her. That he has never loved anyone else like her, ever. That he will never love anyone else. He will tell her that he will fight for her. In fact, he would love to fight for her because he can then fight and love—his two most favorite pastimes.

He will persuade, entice, flatter, beg even, and shower her with gifts, if he thinks that he will be able to "drive."

And the next day, or next week, she might wait to hear from him. But she might find out later that he's texting another girl, dating someone else, and swearing that she is the most beautiful girl in the world. And that he loves her, and will fight for her, and give her the "best of fruits, the tenderest deer, the finest meats that roam the jungle." And the previous woman will be angry and upset. She'll be so shocked that he would dare say the same thing to another girl.

But she should understand that he meant what he said to her and means it with this new girl too. He's just an unripe mango that needs a little more time.

I can see why women are frustrated at man-goes. But look at the alternative. Consider men without a sex drive. They would all be walking around in flip-flops and shorts, some hung over from the party after the

B. D. Foley

rugby game, toothless from fights, laughing about fart jokes, and eating barking pigs, all the time, every day, for the rest of their lives. Without a sex drive, a man would never see the need to straighten up for a lady, to behave, or even think about wearing a suit. And passion fruit? Forget about it.

NOTES

1. Mango.org.

22

Terminating Mr. Wrong

While I was serving overseas, a Russian officer of the KGB (now called the SVR) targeted me for recruitment, as I was targeting him. During one conversation, he mentioned, subtly (there's that word again), that he was hoping to purchase a vehicle from someone in the diplomatic community. He asked me for a copy of the weekly American Embassy newsletter, which often listed vehicles that were for sale. I questioned him, politely, about what kind of vehicle he was interested in, and promised to let him know if such a vehicle came up for sale. Seeing that his first ruse didn't work, Ivan (let's call him) claimed that he was also interested in appliances and requested the newsletter again. I asked him what kind of appliance he needed, and repeated that I would call him if one became available.

Surprise, Ivan was not really interested in purchasing a vehicle or a toaster. What he really wanted were secret documents from the US government. The newsletter, which was an unclassified but sensitive document, was just a subtle way for him to find out if I was pliable.

He tried another tack, in between my attempts to recruit him. One evening he brought up his beautiful *dacha* (a Russian second home) in the countryside on the outskirts of Moscow and even described the size of his plot of land—in square meters. He was hoping to see a reaction, maybe see my eyes "light up" at the mention of property or wealth (and he was also letting me know that he was comfortable in his life and not recruitable).

I simply told him that we measured our real estate in America in "square acres," not meters. He got the message that I was not recruitable, and that was that. Forget about it.

As we know, a sexual predator will often follow a similarly subtle approach as a KGB officer. When I was being targeted by Ivan, above, I was already alert. I also knew who he was, because I had seen him stalking others during parties and diplomatic functions. I recognized his MO (*modus operandi*), both from training and from seeing him in action. When he asked for the newsletter, I already knew exactly what he wanted.

Because I was alert—and not vulnerable—I was able to avoid a serious mistake. And I am not serving in a super-max prison, like my former colleagues Aldrich Ames or James Nicholson.

A young woman can be similarly alert to an offer from someone she knows is targeting her, such as a classmate or coworker. She should politely decline the invitation, with honesty. She can tell him, "Oh, no thanks. I'm seeing someone else." She can say, "No thanks, I'd rather not." She doesn't owe this "Ivan" any elaborate explanation. She's not required to provide her week's or month's schedule. She doesn't need to tell him that she's doing her laundry that night or washing her hair. She can just be honest, firm, and polite.

If this "Ivan" decides to persist, insist, or crosses a line into sexual harassment and becomes a predator, then she must also escalate her response. In the CIA, if an officer is "pitched" by a member of a hostile intelligence organization, she is trained to firmly decline the offer and advise that she will report it. Most schools and businesses have similar procedures for handling sexual harassment. At the least, a young woman needs to firmly decline, tell him to stop the unwanted advances, and inform the harasser that she will report it to school officials or to her supervisor at work. This will usually end it. If he continues, then she should proceed by reporting the behavior immediately.

Not all unwanted advances, however, are from sexual predators. A young woman might be asked out by a nice young man with good intentions—even a prince, but not the prince whom she wants to date, for whatever the reason. But many women have a hard time declining a date, often because they feel compassion (there's that word again) for his feelings.

Sadly, by not wanting to hurt his feelings, a young lady might damage them even more by going out with him. A "pity" date will often send mixed signals, causing him to get his hopes up and leading to worse pain in the future—for both of them.

I wonder about the high number of dates that women of the world have accepted over the centuries because they wanted to be nice, didn't want to hurt a man's feelings, or just couldn't say no. Is the number in the millions or billions? That's also a lot of tickets for seats to watch the gladiators, chariot races, and modern movies. And a lot of wasted time, money, and heartache.

Carly Wisel listed some effective ways to decline a date, in the nicest, least painful way possible:

1. **Be Honest.** Don't lie about a fake boyfriend or your weekend plans. "Express that you're flattered, but not interested. . . . Never say yes just because you feel guilty. You're in no way obligated to go on a date with anybody else! Being turned down right off the bat may be a tougher pill to swallow initially, but it's a better move than to waste both your time and lead someone (who you may very well care about, albeit in a platonic way) on."

2. **Try a "compliment sandwich."** "The best way to let down a friend or someone you already know is to couch your response between kind, truthful compliments. . . . Say something like, 'I have so much fun when I'm with you, but I don't see a romantic future for us. You're hilarious and so sweet, and I'd love to continue our friendship.' Friend zone him, with a sandwich!

3. **Keep the confidence.** Don't publicize his invitation to all of your friends or make fun of him. Wisel advises, "If you're asked out on Facebook or in an email, don't screenshot the exchange or forward the message to your classmates. Everyone's bound to be in this position at some point, and isn't it pretty brave (and flattering) that someone put themselves out there for you?" Respect him.

4. **Talk.** "If someone asks you out through a text, pick up the phone and call them—or go a step further and let the other person know your answer in person." Men should know to ask a girl on a date over the phone or in person—not via texting. Women should know to decline a date in the same way—not via texting. Wise adds that "this will do away with any, 'But what will I do when I see him next?' dread on both ends."

5. **Know why you say no.** Wisel advises a young woman to ask herself why she is declining: Is it based upon gossip or rumors? Is

it because of his "social status"? She explains, "If that's the case, it's likely worth giving them a shot, so assess the real reason and proceed accordingly."[1]

I might add one more suggestion in turning down a man: try a little humor. Awkward situations can often be avoided with a little dash of humor. The American writer E. B. White once declined an invitation by writing, "I must decline, for secret reasons." What man wouldn't smile at that response from a woman?

Last, if it's someone whom you might want to date, but are still undecided: rather than give him your phone number, ask for his. You can then maintain control of the situation. You call the shots. You can decide to call him in the future or not.

And not all relationships work out. Actually, most do not. So it's important that you learn how to break off a relationship amicably. It's called "fired" in employment settings. In espionage it's called "termination."

Termination of a source in the CIA can be risky, even dangerous, especially if he threatens to report it to his government. There are numerous instances where a source has wanted the relationship to continue, whether for money or other reasons. Some of my sources were angry; others were relieved that it was over. One former colleague in the CIA shared that he had a particularly difficult termination: "The source begged, cried, and made all kinds of promises, wildly unrealistic and imaginative claims about how he was going to get this or that information."

Terminating a social relationship can be just as difficult, especially for a woman. I suppose that most women are too caring to approach it cavalierly or carelessly (as men often do). So often a women finds herself feeling guilty or sorry for the young man, who might be begging, crying, and making "all kinds of promises."

I wonder how many women have married a man whom they were unable to stop dating, or terminate, over the centuries. How many women give in to the begging or pressure he might exert on her to keep dating and surrender to his insistence or to her own compassion?

Sources in the CIA are terminated according to certain standards. A young woman can terminate a relationship by following the same considerations:

How? In most cases, except in certain situations where he displays inappropriate or violent behavior, it's best to avoid breakups over text, telephone, or Twitter. She needs to talk to him in person, just as she does when declining a date (above). My brother was dumped by the same woman two times, via text messages, within a month. That's just wrong. Knowing how inconsiderate she is, I think he was lucky; if the relationship had continued, she might have ended up divorcing him over Instagram.

Where? Plan where you're going to say it. If he's emotional, manipulative, or volatile, then you need to do it in a public area: a restaurant, café, or in your home living room, with your Dad sitting across the room, wearing his lavalava.

According to Grant Corser, the Associate Professor of Psychology at Southern Utah University, men will often become aggressive when their goals are blocked or their dating objectives don't work out.[2] When a relative of mine broke up with a boyfriend, he persuaded her to go for one last drive, out in the desert. During the ride, he would not accept "no" for an answer. When he finally realized that the relationship was really finished, he began to yell at her, cursing and calling her vulgar names. He eventually struck her in the face and broke her jaw.

If there's any hint, at all, that a young man has this kind of unstable personality, then the young lady should carefully select where she will inform him that the relationship is over. She might consider having friends or family close by, in an adjacent room or lobby, for instance. Just having others in the vicinity might be enough to preempt any emotional or violent outbursts on his part.

What to say? Third, decide what you are going to say. The young woman who has decided to move on needs to be:

1. Fair. Be honest, but not harsh. Let him down easily. She should not feel compelled to explain why she no longer wants to see him: because he is unattractive, is boring, has a vulgar sense of humor, or has unruly nose hair. Some men will beg to know why she is moving on, but it's just not necessary for her to point out why she no longer wants to see him. "I am just not into you" might be the best message, but worded more subtly: "You're a nice guy, but I don't want to pursue this relationship any further." "It just doesn't feel right."

Dishonest answers will not help. If she tells him "I'm just not ready for a committed relationship at this point in my life," he will most likely decide to wait around until she is ready. And truthfully, she probably wants to be in a committed relationship, just not with him. If she says that she "needs space" or "time," then he will probably just give her both, with the expectation that he will soon be back in the game; he will just be patient until she is ready. Sometimes, simply promising to "remain friends" can cause a persistent man—and they can be very persistent—to hang around. He might just settle for that friend level, reasoning that he will soon convince her that they are more than that and she will someday realize it when she just gets to know him better.

2. Be firm. She needs to avoid waffling, especially if he is trying to negotiate and suggests, "Okay, let's just scale it back and just see each other once a week," "Let's have a temporary separation," or "Let's just go to the concert, since I already have tickets." No, no, and no. Be firm. Stick with your feelings and good judgment.

It's not necessary for you to tell a boyfriend, "You are fired!" like Donald Trump. But be decisive, unyielding, and adamant. Once you have made up your mind, stick with it. You'll be grateful that you did.

3. Be final. He has to know that you're moving on, and he needs to do the same. You're not going to date him again in a month, a year, when he changes his bad behavior, after Christmas, or before the end of the world. He needs to know the truth in order for you to move on and because he needs to get on with his life as well.

Don't keep him hanging. Don't let him hope to see you again, because he will hang on to that hope. Tell him you're sorry but that you know he'll be fine, that you had shared good times together, and that you wish him well for his future. Period.

An article in Buzzfeed by Rianna Rebolinin and Katie Heaney lists the ten worst things to say during a breakup, one of which is "I still care about you." They note that "Saying too many nice or seemingly romantic things during a breakup can be confusing. Compliments don't soften the blow, they twist the knife."[3]

A hurt, determined young man will grasp at any carrot of hope a girl dangles in front of him. A young woman who gives a would-be suitor or her soon-to-be-ex any hope, although well intentioned, is actually doing him more harm than good. She is only encouraging him to believe that they will get back together—someday, somehow—if he just tries hard enough and puts his life on hold until he figures how to get her back. This feeling of caring, of compassion on the girl's part, will just prolong his agony for months rather than days. Don't let him agonize. Don't twist the knife. Let him get on with his life and you can get on with yours. Terminate him.

In extreme cases, a young man will attempt to dramatize the breakup, maybe threaten a new boyfriend or threaten to commit suicide. A member of my basketball team threatened to end his life when his girlfriend announced that she wanted to end the relationship. He locked himself in her bathroom, screaming through the closed door that he was going to kill himself. This kind of behavior is just all the more reason to leave him as soon as possible.

A young man who threatens suicide is merely abusing the young woman. He is using psychological abuse, or emotional blackmail, to exert more pressure on her. She should tell a parent, friend, school counselor, or anyone that she trusts that he is causing her trouble.

In the case of teammate's girlfriend, she did just that. She called us, her friends, and asked that we come over to her home. When we arrived and he heard us, and he realized that she was surrounded by friends, he quickly realized that the drama was not working, and he probably felt a bit silly. He exited the bathroom and went home, and the drama and relationship were both over.

If he continues, however, to threaten her, himself, or others, then she can threaten to call the police and then should follow through with a call if he continues his abusive threats.

Terminating an asset in the CIA is not easy. I found it difficult to cut some sources loose. I was fond of them. We went through a lot together. We even risked our lives together. Breaking up with a boyfriend, no matter the duration of the relationship, can be just as difficult, sad, and stressful. But following the above steps will certainly help a young woman handle it appropriately.

So terminate him.

How to decline a date from a persistent stranger or creep:

1. Firmly say no thanks.
2. Tell him you are not interested and to stop further advances
3. Tell him you will report it if he continues.

How to decline a date:

1. Be honest.
2. Use a compliment sandwich.
3. Be respectful; do not mock him on the Internet.
4. Decline on the phone, or in person, not texting.

5. Know why you are declining.
6. Ask for his phone number rather than give yours.

How to break up with a boyfriend:

1. Let him know your decision in person.
2. Tell him in a safe environment.
3. Be firm.
4. Be fair.
5. Be final.

NOTES

1. Carlye Wisel, "How to Say No to a Date (in the Nicest, Least Painful Way Possible," November 5, 2013, http://www.teenvogue.com/story/how-to-say-no-to-a-date.

2. Grant Corser, interview with the author, February 2015.

3. Ariana Rebolini, and Katie Heaney, "The 10 Worst Things to Say During a Break-up," May 7, 2014, http://www.buzzfeed.com/ariannarebolini/the-10-worst-things-to-say-during-a-break-up#.ogvNzgQ9O.

23
Recruiting
Mr. Right

Once a young lady has avoided, or terminated, Mr. Wrong, it's often a challenge to spot, assess, develop, and recruit Mr. Right. Recent Pew Research has noted that "the share of American adults who have never been married is at an historic high." Young people are getting married later or not at all; in 2014, only 53 percent of never-married adults say that they would like to marry eventually.

The study also concluded that the labor market is a huge hurdle to marriage. "In 1960, 98% of men ages 25 to 34 were in the labor force; by 2012 that share had fallen to 82%." That's 18% of the men who are unemployed.[1]

No wonder that 78 percent of women list "steady job" as the first trait they are looking for in a man. Yes, they want an employed man more than bulging biceps, dreamy eyes, or a six-pack. They want him to have a steady job. They wish for financial security for themselves and their children.

That is what women want in a mate, at least when they reach marrying age. So why all the focus on bulging biceps, dreamy eyes, and six-packs? According to my research, which is not quite as accurate as Pew's, 60 to 90 percent of women are wasting a lot of their time on a young man's looks. If a woman is going to choose a man who has a steady job and is financially stable, then she should start looking for him now. She should stop looking for a stud and start looking for a stud-ent who likes to stud-y.

While I did mention in chapter 1 that this is not another book on how to catch a guy, it's necessary to point out how a young lady can ultimately end up with a young man who is compatible, honorable, and a good match. And a young lady can use the same recruitment cycle we discussed earlier: spot, assess, develop, and recruit or terminate.

Some young ladies might feel that they can sit idly by while men pick and choose, sorting through all the women like CDs in a music store. But she can take an active, proactive role in the recruitment process, and sort and sift through the men. She can sift out the Gweebi's and then meet, greet, and recruit a Gweegi, or Guy With Good Intentions. (I worked in the government way too long; they have an acronym for everything.)

Everyone goes through this same cycle in relationships, which can take hours, days, or months. It's a process, and unfortunately, there is no app for that. Wouldn't it be nice if there were a "Sift the Sap App"? It sure would save time. I would buy that app for my daughter.

Early on in my career at the CIA, I was walking through the headquarters cafeteria and spotted a beautiful young staffer. She had it all: toned figure, big hair (it was the eighties), and a sun tan even in January. She was gorgeous. I arranged to meet her and we went out. During the date, however, I quickly learned that we had absolutely nothing in common. Not walks on the beach. Not getting caught in the rain. Nothing. All she talked about was where she worked out, where she partied, and where she tanned (at her favorite tanning salon).

I actually found myself pleading in my head during our date: *Please, please, this cannot be happening! Nobody this gorgeous can be this shallow! Please have a personality somewhere under all that hair!*

Well, I couldn't find one, at least not one that I was looking for. We finished dinner, and I took her home after about an hour and a half. It was probably the shortest date of my life. It was just too painful. Funny thing—the next day, a colleague told me that he passed her in the hallway of CIA headquarters, chatting with friends at the soda machines. As he walked by the group, he overheard her complain, "You won't believe it. I went out with this guy last night, and it was the most boring date of my life."

Romance is a process, and sometimes it's messy. It can often feel like a total waste of time, effort, and money. But we can at least bring some semblance of order or efficiency to the process. And after all, it is our life, happiness, and future well-being that we are talking about.

There are steps we can take to recruit a spy (and a boyfriend):

1. Spotting. As we discussed earlier, the first step in the recruitment process is spotting. Intelligence officers must first find sources, so they need to go where the sources hang out. They frequent almost any kind of gathering to locate potential sources, introduce themselves, and begin a relationship. Ladies should be as determined in their search for a potential spouse.

Susan A. Patton, who came to be known as the "Princeton Mom," wrote an interesting letter to the editor of the *Daily Princetonian* in 2013 regarding the need for women to find a husband while they are in college, specifically at Princeton. She noted,

> When I was an undergraduate in the mid-seventies, the 200 pioneer women in my class would talk about navigating the virile plains of Princeton as a precursor to professional success. Never being one to shy away from expressing an unpopular opinion, I said that I wanted to get married and have children. It was seen as heresy.
>
> For most of you, the cornerstone of your future and happiness will be inextricably linked to the man you marry, and you will never again have this concentration of men who are worthy of you.
>
> Here's what nobody is telling you: Find a husband on campus before you graduate.[2]

I was lucky. I attended a private university with fifteen thousand fabulous female students and did not marry one of them. As the years passed after graduation, the pool shrunk exponentially. By the time I was thirty, most, if not all, of the women I had dated or wanted to date were married, with children. The pool of fifteen thousand potential mates had drastically dried up. (Lucky for me there was one pool left, a swimming pool at the Okapi Hotel in Africa!)

While Mrs. Patton took a lot of heat for suggesting that young women find a husband while in college, she was merely stating the obvious. Women will never again find such a "concentration of men who are worthy." Sure, it's always possible to find someone outside the college environment. But she will never, ever be in such a target-rich environment again.

As an intelligence officer overseas, I frequented mainly diplomatic functions, but also seminars, art exhibits, business luncheons, basketball games, and banquets, almost nightly. After my day job, my night job consisted of going to parties. The gatherings provided the venue to fish for sources. Once there, it was up to me to meet as many as I could.

I mostly hunted hard targets: Russians, Chinese, and Iranians. And it was not easy to locate them in huge crowds, often numbering in the hundreds. I had to introduce myself quickly, ascertain whether the person was someone interesting or not, and continue the conversation or excuse myself quickly. Time was short. I often went home with a handful of business cards, most from someone in this or that association or organization or think-tank who was looking to network.

I slowly learned how to maximize my time. As I mentioned, I often took my wife along to assist in spotting. I noticed that certain groups of people would congregate in certain areas of the hall. Russians would inevitably hover around the smoked salmon and caviar, and I would introduce myself in between bites. They love salmon.

A supervisor often counseled me to "cut a swath" when I attended these parties. I had to meet as many as possible. To spot a good young man, a young lady needs to attend social events, activities, and mix and mingle.

Ladies, cut a swath. Be proactive and assertive.

2. Assessing. Next comes assessing, or judging, a person. Once I had met a potential target in my CIA work, I needed to assess him. I needed to ascertain if he was someone with access, vulnerabilities, intelligence, the right demeanor. Did he warrant further developing?

A young lady often assesses a young man instinctively. Once she has met a young man, she will make a whole series of snap judgments: Is he handsome? Is he friendly? Is he smart? Does he floss? Does he polish his shoes? (Young men, are you still reading this, after I told you this book is not for you? Well, if you are, then floss and polish your shoes.). She will decide in a few minutes whether he's someone she would like to get to know better, accept a date with, or excuse herself quickly. Fortunately, she has more time than a typical operations officer at a diplomatic function.

Once a woman has spotted someone that she's interested in, and assessed him enough to know that she would like to see more of him, the next steps are important.

- Don't be in a rush to say yes, or *oui*, in my wife's case. During a recent episode of *American Pickers*, I heard Mike comment, when he saw an old Airstream trailer, which he always wanted, "I didn't let on that I was interested." At another point, he noted, "Don't show your cards up front." Women should talk to a man like they are negotiating for an Airstream trailer, or playing cards. It is not necessary to let on that she is extremely interested in him. She can simply pause for a second or two, mentally check her calendar, maybe tell him, "I don't know if I can go tomorrow." Like I said before, make him work a bit. Keep him on his toes. Make him appreciate you. I'm not saying to play "hard to get." I'm saying to be hard to get.

- Don't be in a rush to give up kisses or too much affection. Men will be happy to take whatever you give them, whenever you give it, for free. But men will often think *why buy the cow when the milk is free?* Men will be happy to take all the affection you can give, for as long as you give it, at no cost to them: no cost in commitment, no cost in investment, and often no cost in respect. Make him invest before you give too much, or before you invest your heart.

3. Developing. If all goes well, the next step is developing the relationship. If she decides that the young man is worth it, she will further the relationship: identify common interests, build rapport and trust, explore his personality, and vet and test him. *Developing* means building rapport and furthering the relationship. Developing also leads to a stronger relationship, going steady, being exclusive, or even marriage. This is when you can start to fall in love, and not before!

A young lady will gradually become quite sure that he has potential, that he is polite and fun and intelligent and that he likes her too. But this stage might also be the most crucial. A couple of tips for the developmental stage:

- During the developmental stage, always end a date on a high-note. Don't end the evening discussing the kidnapping of Nigerian girls or beheadings by ISIS in Iraq or the death of a friend's grandmother. Always end a date on a positive, uplifting, happy note because that is what he will remember until he sees you again—which might be a day, or a week, or a month. Don't let him dwell on a negative last impression. Rather, let him think about a wonderful conversation about skiing or travel to Europe or daisies or unicorns. You want him to have pleasant thoughts when he thinks about you, right up until he sees you again. As a CIA officer, I knew that I might not see a source for months, or even longer, and I wanted him to have positive thoughts about me for that period of time. A young woman wants a man to have similar positive thoughts about her until he sees her again.

- Create a magic moment, or two, during the date. Participate in a special activity, or create a unique moment: push him into the water fountain, run through a park in the rain, have a mini-food fight, spray him with Silly String, go ice-blocking down a grassy slope, tell him a joke while he's drinking his milk. Magic moments are memories. They are memories that you will both cherish, maybe for the next twenty-five years, or longer. Magic moments, which become magic memories, will deepen and enrich the relationship.

- Bring up past conversations from previous dates, and allow him to recount something important, maybe something that occurred during a magic moment, such as how much he cares for you: "Do you remember when we went for that walk along the beach and you said . . ." Coaxing, or allowing, your boyfriend to describe a wonderful date you enjoyed, and the conversation, actually allows him to replay it in his mango mind. It refreshes the magic moment. It dusts off the cobwebs. It's interesting psychology, and it works. It works with sources, and it will work with him.

A young woman should look to actively recruit Mr. Right. She should be as vigilant, intuitive, watchful, and careful as an operations officer, or an employment specialist. She can be as proactive and assertive as a headhunter at an employment agency. So, girls, be headhunters!

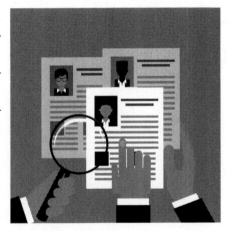

1. Spot him.
2. Assess him.
3. Develop him.
4. Always end a date on a positive note.
5. Make magic moments.
6. Recruit him.

NOTES

1. Wendy Wang and Kim Parker, "Record Share of Americans Have Never Married," September 24, 2014, http://www.pewsocialtrends.org/2014/09/24/record-share-of-americans-have-never-married/.

2. Susan A Patton, "Letter to the Editor," Dailyprincetoninan.com, March 29, 2013.

24

Training Mr. Right

Let's face it. Men are all a work in progress. They are all evolving or devolving, all heading in one direction or the other on the evolutionary scale or cycle.

One day, after a date with a former girlfriend, years ago, I was cleaning under the seats of my vehicle and found a spiral notebook. I didn't recognize it as mine and opened it, only to find she had written my name at the top of one page, with pros and cons lists of words underneath. Unfortunately for me, the cons list was longer. But I found hope in the fact that she had written one word under the pros column—*potential*.

I remember an elementary teacher had once used the same word to describe me in a report card: "shows potential." All men show some kind of potential. But how to judge if a man has potential and has any chance of reaching it?

Men have the potential to be honest.
Men have the potential to be responsible.
Men have the potential to be caring.
Men have the potential to be cheerful.

Reliable, stable, calm, unflappable, ambitious. All qualities that anyone can attain—that anyone has the potential to reach.

But not all do. At least not yet; not until they are ripe.

It must be 99.99 percent of men who do not reach their full potential.

I know that I have not, and I am grateful that my wife is still helping me, still training me, coaching, and hoping that I will at least get close. And I hope that her Pros and Cons list is at least a little more balanced.

So how can a young woman help a good young man reach his potential? How to convince him to wear socks and to floss?

First of all, a young lady can set the bar—like the bar of a high jump. She can set the standards—the expectations—from the outset, from the very first date. She might not know it, but a young lady can tell a young man when to jump and how high and, more important, when not to jump.

She can encourage wholesome activities instead of make-out sessions. Ballet or mixed martial arts? Parking and sparking, or ice-blocking and sidewalk chalking? A young lady has more influence than she might think. If a young woman only knew her true power, then the men of the world would be looking to be empowered and not vice versa.

While serving in Afghanistan, a US military unit stopped by our compound to dust off, get some drinking water, and use our bathroom, which was literally a hole in the mud wall but was still better than the conditions they encountered on the road. One soldier of the unit was a female, and as she walked through the courtyard, we all stopped in our tracks to stare. We had not seen a lady in months, and we were all in awe. I truly believe that most of the men felt more fascination than lust. Maybe I would call it wonder.

In hindsight, I know that it was just nice to have a woman around. It was nice to see a woman, even if she was dressed in boots and dusty fatigues. What a dreadful world it would be without women.

And what a wonderful world with empowered women! What a wonderful world with women who insist on standards, on values, on men reaching the bar. And her insistence actually helps a young man reach his potential, helps him "ripen" from boy to man to gentleman. Her insistence makes all the difference for herself and for him.

And although he might not reach his full potential with her, he'll be closer to it when he meets some other lady in his future. He'll be the wiser and all the more gentlemanly. And the next girlfriend should thank the first for passing on a better man!

While attending college in Hawaii, I became interested in a young woman from the Philippines—Susan, a fellow student. She was a beautiful young woman, very refined and ladylike.

I asked her to the prom about a month away. Not a week later, I noticed another beauty on campus. I asked this girl out on a date as well. (Yes, I did that.) Soon, Susan heard about it (did she have sources?) and approached me while I was walking to class. She informed me that she had learned I had dated another young woman, and she had decided that she could no longer accept my invitation to the prom. When I expressed shock at her decision, she explained that in her culture, a woman had many male "suitors," but not vice versa. She had standards, or a bar, to which she expected men to reach.

Although I still acted somewhat like a "dog in a field full of rabbits," as my dad referred to me, and still "chased" girls during the ensuing years, I was much more cognizant of my actions and of what women must feel when they see us dogs running around. I'm grateful for Susan's training.

Girls can help train men to be:

1. Honest. She can insist that he tell the truth, always. She can let him know that she does not tolerate "little white lies," or lies of any color. She can let him know that she does not stand for fabrications, even exaggerations. She can train him to be honest at all costs. And she can tell him that she appreciates his honesty when he is staying up too late at night, sleeping late in the morning, missing class, or eating the dorm mother's barking pig.

A favorite story of mine on honesty was told by James Herriott, author of *All Creatures Great and Small* and a series of books about his life as a veterinarian in Great Britain, which was later made into a TV series. During one episode, a farmer's wife presents his partner, Siegfried Farnon, with a piece of cake to "test," wanting his approval. Little did he know, however, she had substituted a neighbor lady's cake, to see if he could tell the difference and to find out if he was truly honest. After tasting it, and a long pause, with the family waiting in anticipation, Siegfried stated, "This is a good cake. It's a very good cake indeed. But, if you'll permit me, I'm bound to say, it's not up to your usual standard." She answers, "What a wonderful man!"

His honesty, especially in a situation that could've backfired on him, was more delicious than the cake. Honesty in the face of that kind of pressure—and potential embarrassment or prosecution—is honesty indeed.

2. Trustworthy. If he constantly shows up late for a date, she can let him know that it's unacceptable. She can let him know that it seems he's not very anxious to see her or he would've been on time. She can insist that they be on time to parties, to school, to work (as she is!). She can tell him that she expects him to be punctual when he's supposed to pick her up at a particular place, at a particular time.

She should make it clear that she expects to trust him in social settings, or camping, fishing, hunting, or hiking. She should emphasize that he is to protect her. If he doesn't agree, then she will have to decide whether she can live for the next fifty years with someone who is not reliable.

3. Polite. Tell him that manners start with the word *man*! She can wait in the car until he goes around and opens the door for her. She can wait by the restaurant door until he opens it. She can refuse to depart her home when he drives up and honks or texts to announce his arrival. She can insist that he meet her parents. And she can train him to be polite to her parents, to her friends, and to his friends.

If he does not accept the training, then she has to decide if it will be worth it living with someone who will never open a door for her nor treat her parents with courtesy. Will it be bearable to live with someone who doesn't know the words *please, thank you, no thank you, excuse me, pardon me,* and *I'm sorry*? One of the biggest lies ever foisted on society was "Love is never having to say you're sorry," ironically, from the movie *Love Story*. Really? I say sorry to my wife a lot because I'm always messing up. That's love.

Will it be worth living with a handsome young man, soon to be an old man, who will not wash a dish, who throws his underwear on the floor, who will not squeegee the shower walls (yes, she has trained me to do that), who refuses to take out the garbage (still training me, but almost there!), and who does not believe in ladies first? Who will not say sorry?

My wife reminds all of us in our family to say thank you to someone who gives you a ride home, to not put our elbows on the table, to sit up straight, and to practice good phone manners. She was raised in the old world—Africa and in Europe, where she was taught old-fashioned manners that we all need to remember.

We try to train our daughter's female friends when they call on the phone and ask, rudely, "Can I speak to your daughter?" without so much as a greeting, introduction, or anything. I regularly stop her friend and say, "Good morning," then pause, then ask who it is, how she's doing, and then coax her to ask me how I am. Pity the foolish boy that calls up for a date and forgets these basic manners.

4. Sociable. As I have mentioned, most men don't like to play dress up. Many men, if given the chance, would stay home and watch their 499 cable TV channels. After all, there's always a rugby, cricket, or curling match to watch in between shooting zombies and space aliens on Xbox while eating Cheetos. I love Cheetos. And chocolate.

But a woman can help men be more sociable, if she is determined. And he will learn to socialize and engage in polite chit-chat, munching, and mingling. And before she even realizes it, he is all shaved, showered, and dressed up at a party, wearing socks, conversing rather then texting with interesting people. And he's sipping rather than gulping his drinks, and selecting hors-d'oeuvres from a tray rather than digging Cheetos from under the cushions of his couch.

If a woman insists, the young man will actually learn to enjoy social- izing, not just to please her but because he enjoys the interaction. He will find that the time socializing affords him opportunities to hold her hand, to enjoy watching her laugh, to appreciate her intelligence and her sense of humor as she converses with friends. He will wonder at how easily she makes new friends. He will see her all over again, through the eyes of her friends, like he did when he first saw her in class or at the party or by the swimming pool.

And he will wait for her to look his way and smile from across the room. (Yes, I do that.) And that smile and those dark eyes, will remind him that he appreciates her more than anything else in the world. Social- izing will give him an opportunity to see her over and over with wonder.

If he's not willing to be trained, then she will have to decide whether she can be married to a man who won't dance with her for the next fifty years. She will have to decide if she can be married to a man who prefers to stay home and watch football rather than go to a wedding reception or holiday party. She might have to decide if she can stand dating a young man who is antisocial or miserable and realize that he will eventually rub off on her and that she might become miserable too.

And people do rub off on each other. When two cars collide, they swap dents and paint. When two people bump enough over the years, they end up sharing mannerisms, personality traits, and quirks. Be aware that you will be wearing his dents and paint as well.

5. Healthy. My wife often tells me, "You've had enough." I could eat every snack or treat in our pantry at a sitting if she didn't stop me. I still raid the pantry when she leaves the house, like some grade-school boy, knowing that she cannot catch me. While the cat is away, the mice will play.

Women can train men to eat their vegetables, to get out of the house, to go to the gym more often, or to visit the gym a little less, to sleep more or sleep less. She can tell him that it's late at night and he has a final exam tomorrow and that there will be plenty of time for kissing tomorrow night after his test!

Young women can train young men in the concept of moderation: eat in moderation, play video games in moderation, cut wood in moderation, buy tools in moderation (yes, I'm learning that), shop in moderation (she is learning that).

6. Spiritual. Every church that I have ever attended, from all denominations, seems to have a larger number of women in attendance. Women just seem to be more in touch with their spiritual side. Take him to church, any church. If he won't go to church, then take him in the woods or to a beautiful waterfall, or library, and help him meditate. Help him understand that there might be something more to life. There might be a God. Help him see that there is more to life than cage-fighting and football. Help him to learn how to look outside himself, to be compassionate to others, to be kind, to show charity. Seeing outside himself, seeing the needs and wishes and others, and understanding others will help him see himself and help him grow as a spiritual being.

7. His best. Many men would probably forget to shave, trim their unruly nose hairs, or bathe if they weren't reminded. My mom was the heart and soul of our home. She kept us all in sync and in harmony as best she could. Our dad relied on her for everything, including giving him an allowance (she handled all the finances), baking rhubarb pies, darning socks (who does that anymore?), and telling him if it was his bath day. Hard to believe that some men still have a bath day. She wanted him to bathe once a day, and he thought that once every three or four days was fine. They compromised on every third day.

We were all heartbroken when she was diagnosed with cancer near the end of a wonderful life. Although our retired military dad tried to cope with the news as best he could, he was devastated. She was the center of his life.

A month before her passing I had returned to our old family home to see her, for the last time. As I sat on my mom's bed, holding her hand, my dad entered the room and asked, "Mary Leone, is today my bath day?" "No, dear, your bath day is tomorrow," she replied.

There she was, fighting cancer for the past five years, very close to dying, and she was still keeping track of his bath day. It might seem silly to some, but she tried her best to train him, to keep him bathed and looking his best, to keep him at his best, until the very end.

Woman can be a man's best friend, his lover, and his confidant, but she can also be his coach. So, girls, be your man's coach, for life.

Help him to be all of these things:

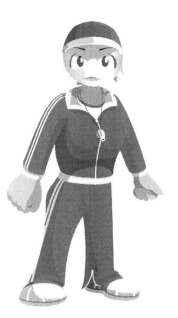

1. Honest
2. Trustworthy
3. Polite
4. Sociable
5. Healthy
6. Spiritual
7. His best

25

Pain and Suffering from Daughters

Can a father sue his daughter for pain and suffering? If so, I imagine that I could get a lot of money. My daughter caused me pain and suffering from the moment she was born.

My wife, Jacqueline, and I were living overseas with our first son during the mid-1990s. We had been waiting five long years for our second child without success. Actually, we weren't just waiting. We tried several remedies—some not so conventional. Friends cautioned against excessive exercise or tight underwear. One told us to take her temperature daily, even have her stand on her head. A doctor we visited during home leave gave even worse advice, after expensive tests: "Well, if it worked once, it will work again; that'll be $300, pay at the desk on your way out."

A US government physician ended up being our lifesaver. He gave us a list of dos and don'ts, which we followed carefully. And miraculously, at the end of the six months, which was his deadline before we were to undergo medical procedures, his guidance had worked, and she was pregnant.

A few months later, we picked up and moved our growing family to another European city. As the happy day approached, we all settled into our apartment and began to adjust to our new life. I began work, my wife found friends, grocery stores, and a farmer's market down the street where she could purchase her fresh fruits and vegetables, and our oldest son began school. We all waited with unimaginable anticipation for the big day.

When she felt contractions one night, we rushed to the hospital located in a rather wealthy suburb. But it turned out to be a "hurry up and wait" situation. We needn't have rushed; we had plenty of time and ended up waiting in a room for the contractions to become more regular and the cervix to dilate. At 11:30 p.m., Jacqueline was finally approaching childbirth, and the hospital staff moved us to the birthing room, where they laid her on the bed and instructed me to don a hospital gown and white slippers.

At around 11:45 p.m., she turned to me and asked me to get the camcorder. I told her that was impossible, reminding her in my kindest voice possible that we had left the camcorder out in the car. Her dark eyes grew darker, and her voice took on a tone of ominous warning.

"Go get the camera!"

"Okay," I reassured her, "I'll go!"

I was mostly afraid that I would miss the event—the birth that we had been waiting for, all those years. To tell you the truth, I don't know why I was anxious to be in the birthing room at all. I never have relished the idea of watching a live childbirth. I often wonder what ever happened to the good ol' days when the father would relax in the waiting room, pace the floor a bit, and maybe read a magazine where it's nice and safe.

I ripped off my slippers and gown, ran out of the obstetrics ward, to the elevator, and down to the ground floor. I exited the elevator and ran past the front desk—hmm, nobody there—and then wham! I bounced off the front glass doors of the hospital. *Strange that the main doors of the hospital are locked*, I thought.

"Hello! Hello!" I shouted. I could not find a soul on this floor of the hospital. In my panic, I could not think of anything else to do but return to the elevator and try another floor. I descended to the basement and entered a dark hallway, where I immediately experienced flashbacks to horror movies of deserted hospitals. I saw the dark silhouette of a man at the other end of the hall, mopping the floor, and I ran to him.

"Excuse me," I blurted out, "can you tell me how to exit the hospital?" He hadn't been in too much of a hurry mopping the floor and was not in any more of a hurry telling me how to get out of there. He slowly turned toward me and propped an elbow on his mop.

"Well," he drawled, "you go to the end of this hall, then take a right, then a left, then follow that hall a little ways to the Emergency Room, and you will find an exit there." I was gone before he had finished the last word and shouted thanks as I was rounding the next corner.

As I exited the emergency wing, I noticed that I was now on a different street than my car, so I had to run around the hospital to the front entrance and out through the parking lot. Our car was parked on the street near the entrance to that parking lot. As I sprinted across the parking lot, I noticed that the entrance was barred with a nine- or ten-foot-high wrought-iron gate. And the guard shack at the entrance was empty. So I did what any crazed, soon-to-be-father-again would do—I jumped up on the gate, grabbed the top rail, pulled myself up, swung my legs over, and dropped. Hey, no problem—I'm invincible!

In a matter of seconds, I had my wife's bag with the video camera inside and was back at the gate. Again thinking, *No problem!* Except now I had a bag with me that I could not throw over the gate, for fear of damaging the camera. I still had an ample supply of adrenaline, however, rushing through my veins. That wonderful substance that inspires you at the arrival of a baby or the police was telling my brain—*Go, dude!* I jumped, grabbed the top rail with one hand, balanced the bag, pulled myself up, swung my legs around, and then sat there, wondering, *What now, dude?*

Before I could even decide my next move, however, it happened. My right leg, which I had rested against the gate, for balance, slipped between the vertical bars. I found myself falling forward, with my leg slipping between the bars and sliding down toward a metal plate, which ran horizontally along the bottom of the gate. And all I could think of was how to save the camcorder.

I should have been thinking about how to save my leg. My right shin impacted first on the edge of the metal plate—kind of like a reverse guillotine. The impact of the metal plate on my right leg caused me to pitch to my left, where I attempted to land on my left foot. But my left foot struck the pavement at such an awkward angle that it rolled over, and I twisted my ankle very badly. And that's where I found myself—face down on the pavement, but with the bag still securely in my hand.

It's an interesting phenomenon that when you stub your toe at night, it takes a second for the pain to reach your brain. Since I'm six foot five inches, I wonder if it sometimes takes longer for the pain to arrive.

I enjoyed the cool pavement on my face for a few moments before I remembered that my wife was giving birth at any minute. I don't really know how, but I made it to my feet, while feeling my left foot swelling in my shoe and blood trickling down my right leg. I just kept telling myself that I couldn't miss the birth.

I began the journey back to the birthing room, retracing my steps through the parking lot and around the hospital, limping on both legs, whining, laughing a bit at the ridiculousness of the situation, but mostly whining. The emergency room attendant watched me enter and told me that he'd call for a doctor immediately. I just put my head down and forged ahead, hopping, skipping, moaning, and explaining as I passed his desk that my wife was having a baby.

"Didn't you forget something? Like your wife?" he chuckled. Oh, that's a good one. Hilarious, just hilarious! A regular Jimmy Kimmel!

I somehow managed to limp through the dark hallways, past the scary mop-man, up the elevator, and back to the birthing room. I tore off my shoes, replaced my slippers and gown, and reached my wife's side just in the nick of time.

As I sat down, I realized that my pain was growing worse by the minute. I even considered requesting an epidural for myself, although I dared tell the nurse earlier that my wife did not need one. (Yes, I said that!) Some men seem so immersed in the whole birthing experience that they even say, "We are pregnant." I certainly felt it at that moment. I decided that I would first try and ease some of the pain by elevating my legs. I knew that technique from Boy Scout first aid—elevate the injured appendage to limit the blood flow and reduce swelling—something like that.

But there was only one set of stirrups, and my wife was using them, so I pulled a chair next to her and propped my two legs on stools positioned on either side of her bed—one alongside and the other under the upraised head of her bed. Jacqueline didn't notice, but the nurses and doctor gave me puzzled looks, obviously wondering why I was in the same position as my wife—legs up and spread—and practicing shallow breathing.

My position probably helped with the swelling and bleeding, but it did nothing for the pain. When Jacqueline turned to me and complained, I responded with a very genuine and heartfelt "I know, honey, I know." We moaned together. We groaned together. Never has a husband been so convincing in feeling his wife's pain, nor been a more sympathetic father. The nurses were quite impressed.

A week later, Jacqueline was still in the hospital. They keep ladies longer there—undoubtedly some European women's conspiracy to avoid returning home and taking care of their starving husbands and children—but I digress. My older son and I made our daily pilgrimage to the hospital to see Mama.

He was missing his mama and growing particularly tired of hot dogs and pork and beans. In his five-year-old mind, it was obviously the baby's fault. On the way home one night, he looked up at me from the passenger seat and asked, "When we go back to America, are we going to take the baby with us?"

"What would you like to do?" I volleyed the question back at him.

"Let's leave her," he replied. He had had enough. His mother had been stolen by the new baby. The baby had broken his heart, along with my shin.

Years later, our baby girl has grown up—and she is still hurting me. We were joking and teasing each other one day after school. She started backing me up by poking me in the tummy with her index finger, teasing. "Don't break your finger on that concrete," I warned her.

"Oh really?" she shot back. "I guess it's just not dry yet."

My little girl still causes me pain from time to time. But I love her. And I'm still full of wonder at how precious she is.

26
Zuzu's Petals

ANOTHER CHAPTER FOR DADS

Daughters need their dads and not just for someone to take her to the daddy/daughter night at school. Dads are an integral part of a daughter's life.

And creeps—including predators, stalkers, and rapists—know that.

An acquaintance, Fabrice, shared some advice: a young lady should never let a boy know that she doesn't have a relationship with her father, brother, or uncle; she should never divulge that she's without a male figure in her life to protect her; and she should never reveal that she's mad at her dad or that she hasn't seen him in ten years. She should keep that to herself, if she can, because a predator will look to exploit any lack of masculine influence, or protection, in her life. Not only that, Fabrice added, "A predator will try to cut any existing ties between a young lady and her father, or to other masculine influences in her life, such as a brother or other relative." A sexual predator will try and isolate her from her support network, especially from men in that network.

A papa is probably the most important member of a young woman's network. He can be her rock. He can be the example of how a man should treat a wife and how a future husband should treat her. He can also give her confidence, hope, and love.

To do that, a papa must be involved in her life. A papa must keep an open line of communication with his daughter, even when she resents it. She is growing up, after all, and might not feel like she needs her dad any longer. It's much easier to help a daughter and to protect her if she has trust and will confide in her papa.

A good friend once told me that a papa needs to go to his daughter's bedroom before she sleeps, sit on the edge of her bed, and tell her he loves her. He should tuck her in until she leaves for college. He should sit on the edge of her bed the same way he did when he told her bedtime stories as a child.

He needs to show her love and attention, the same way that George Bailey did in the movie *It's a Wonderful Life* (my papa's favorite movie). In a wonderful scene from the movie, George sits beside his daughter Zuzu and comforts her after petals have fallen off her rose. He pretends to paste the petals back on but secretly put the petals in his pants pocket. He also lays his hand on her curly hair and wonders at how precious she is—more precious than anything.

A papa needs to sit on his maturing daughter's bed as well and tell her it's her turn to tell bedtime stories. He needs to encourage her to tell him about her day. And if she hesitates, then he needs to elicit stories from her. He needs to use spy skills on her.

By the way, the anesthesia they use on teenagers while having their wisdom teeth pulled is wonderful, and it lasts a long time; it is better than any "truth serum." I got names and I got places, even using direct questions! It was the easiest interrogation I have ever done!

But if he doesn't have anesthesia, he can use the same elicitation ploys that she uses on boys: give to get ("Honey, you wouldn't believe what happened to me at the office"), you-me-same-same ("Oh my, that happened to me too in high school years ago"), assumption ("I bet you did very well on that math exam"), flattery ("I'm so proud of your grades in school, how considerate you are to your brother, and how helpful you have been with your mother"), and current events ("Did you hear about the hurricane in the Southern States?").

A papa can use spy skills on her to open lines of communication, to develop rapport, to build her confidence, to show her love, and to empower her.

And a papa needs to tell his daughter often that he loves her. If he's uncomfortable telling his daughter that he loves her, then he could start the habit in the family. My dad was not very expressive until my younger brother decided to soften him up by telling him, "Good night. I love you," one night before going to bed. My dad was uncomfortable at first, and coughed and mumbled a bit, but he actually began saying it to us too. And he told us for the rest of his life. Old dogs can learn new tricks.

Girls need to hear the words *I love you*. But there's another magic phrase besides "I love you." It's a magic phrase that I don't use nearly enough but have been trying to say more often. It's a phrase that can stop fights, heal hurt feelings, and soothe concerns. It's a simple but magic phrase that can open lines of communication, especially between a dad and daughter or mother and daughter or brother and daughter. It's . . . wait for it . . . "I understand why you feel that way," or "I understand why you are upset." They both start with *I understand.*

More than anything, women want to know that they are understood. Women want to feel understood even more than they want to feel right, or win the argument (which they really love!). Most of the arguments I have had with my wife could've been shortened to a few seconds, instead of hours or days if I had merely replied, "I understand why you are so upset." I understand why you feel pent up at home, bored with the same chores day in and day out. I understand why you miss your parents in Africa and your sisters in Europe. I understand why you're frustrated, sad, scared, and upset when our older son marries a foreigner (yes, she really said that), nervous when our younger son is playing his trumpet at the concert or when our daughter is in a basketball game. I understand, which implies "I sympathize."

Women want to know that we do not just see them, but we also feel their emotions. And more important, they want to know that we're making an effort to feel them.

I shared this secret with a nephew who was in trouble with his mom, my sister. He had burned holes in their new trampoline tarp with fireworks, and she was furious at his carelessness and subsequent lack of caring. I told him to try the magic line, "I understand why you are upset at me." And I advised him to tell her how he would fix the holes. But I added, most important, that he must really mean what he says. Miraculously, he tried it, and it worked. He was out of the doghouse!

So dads and moms, tell your daughter that you understand why she's upset or disappointed or unhappy, that it was really a rough day, and reassure her that tomorrow will be better; the sun will come up, time will heal, she will fall in love again, she will find a good and real man someday, unlike the fool she once dated.

Tell her you will always protect her so other fools do not hurt her. There's a popular song, at least to young men, that goes like this:

Can I have your daughter for the rest of my life?
Say yes, say yes 'cause I need to know.

You say I'll never get your blessing to 'til the day I die,
Tough luck, my friend, but the answer is no!
Why you gotta be so rude?
Don't you know I'm human too?
Why you gotta be so rude?
I'm gonna marry her anyway.[1]

A father and composer, Benji Cowart, heard the above lyrics and reacted as most fathers would. No one likes to hear someone say that some young man is going to take his daughter anyway. So Benji wrote his own "Rude" response, called "The Dad's Side of the Story." Here are a few lines:

Get back in your Pinto. It's time that you go. The answer is no.
You say you want my daughter for the rest of your life,
well, you gotta make more than burgers and fries.
Get out your momma's basement, go and get you a life.
Son, you're twenty-eight, don't you think it's time?
Why you gotta call me rude? I'm doing what a dad should do—
keep her from a fool like you.[2]

This dad's response might seem a little harsh at first glance. This singing dad talks about punching the young man's face, and making him "go away." While he probably wrote the words in jest, this dad is obviously not going to sit idly by while some fool targets his daughter. He plans to protect her.

But you can tell your daughter that she needs to also protect herself until that real man—the right man—comes along. Convince her. Bribe her if you have to. I offered my daughter one hundred dollars if she would not kiss a boy before her sixteenth birthday and two hundred if she made it to seventeen. She made it to both birthdays, probably because she didn't find a boy worth losing a few hundred dollars over. I imagine I will pay a boy to kiss her before her eighteenth birthday.

And last, young men, if any of you have actually read this far, after I told you that this book is not for you—rest assured that we know you will be watching our daughters. But our daughters, now secret agent women with spy skills, will be watching you right back. Actually, they will be surveilling you, assessing you, eliciting information from you, and then terminating you.

And us papas (and mamas), we will be watching you too.

NOTES

1.   Magic!, "Rude," accessed September 9, 2015, http://www.metrolyrics.com/rude-lyrics-magic.html.

2.   Benji and Jenna Coward, "Magic! 'Rude' Parody (The Dad's Side of the Story)"; July 10, 2014, https://www.youtube.com/watch?v=TzyQx6AL1MQ.

Afterword

Women who have been harmed by boyfriends, husbands, or predators can leave abusive relationships, avoid bad men in the future, and eventually find love with a good and real man. I am happy to see that Elizabeth Smart, once a victim, has found love and happiness in a happy marriage. During an interview, years after her kidnapping, Elizabeth noted, "Nobody is trial-free, but we have a choice. We can choose to allow our experiences to hold us back, and to not allow us to become great or achieve greatness in this life. Or we can allow our experiences to push us forward, to make us grateful for every day we have and to be all the more thankful for those who are around us."

Elizabeth added that her mother counseled her, "The best punishment you could ever give him (her attacker) is to be happy." And Elizabeth remarked, "And that's exactly what I'm trying to do for the rest of my life, is be happy."[1]

If you have been a target or victim of abuse, it's not too late for you to be happy. You don't have to continue to suffer in other abusive relationships. And a young woman doesn't have to stay in a destructive relationship. She doesn't have to continue being abused or being a victim. She can choose a new life and choose the path of happiness.

Therapy or counseling is always a beneficial, wonderful means to recovery as well; therapy can greatly help a young woman unburden herself of any unwarranted guilt she might feel or pain or self-destructive thoughts.

And a young man doesn't have to continue being a predator. He doesn't have to continue to be a stalker or manipulator. He can decide to

B. D. Foley

treat women like they deserve to be treated: as precious daughters, with respect and with kindness. He can choose who he wants to be.

In spy circles, we sometimes referred to the process of espionage, or spying, as a dance. I worked to persuade targets to provide intelligence, to do the "espionage dance." If a target refused to become a source, we often said that he just "did not want to dance."

Young men can stop doing the dance of manipulation, deceit, and abuse. Young men do not have to continue to be predators, targeting women.

And young women do not have to continue doing the dance either, that dance of abuse. It's not too late. It's never too late.

> 'Twas battered and scarred, and the auctioneer
> Thought it scarcely worth his while
> To waste much time on the old violin,
> But held it up with a smile:
> "What am I bidden, good folks," he cried,
> "Who'll start the bidding for me?"
> "A dollar, a dollar"; then, "Two!" "Only two?
> Two dollars, and who'll make it three?
> Three dollars, once; three dollars, twice;
> Going for three—" But no,
> From the room, far back, a gray-haired man
> Came forward and picked up the bow;
> Then, wiping the dust from the old violin,
> And tightening the loose strings,
> He played a melody pure and sweet
> As a caroling angel sings.
> The music ceased, and the auctioneer,
> With a voice that was quiet and low,
> Said: "What am I bid for the old violin?"
> And he held it up with the bow.
> "A thousand dollars, and who'll make it two?
> Two thousand! And who'll make it three?
> Three thousand, once, three thousand, twice,
> And going, and gone," said he.
> The people cheered, but some of them cried,
> "We do not quite understand
> What changed its worth." Swift came the reply:
> "The touch of a master's hand."
> And many a man with life out of tune,

And battered and scarred with sin,
Is auctioned cheap to the thoughtless crowd,
Much like the old violin.
A "mess of pottage," a glass of wine;
A game—and he travels on.
He is "going" once, and "going" twice,
He's "going" and almost "gone."
But the Master comes, and the foolish crowd
Never can quite understand
The worth of a soul and the change that's wrought
By the touch of the Master's hand.[2]

NOTES

1. Stephanie Grimes, "Elizabeth Smart: 'The best punishment I could give him is to be Happy,'" April 11, 2012, http://www.ksl.com/?sid=19942794.

2. Myra Brooks, "Touch of the Master's Hand."

About the Author

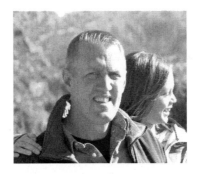

B. D. FOLEY is a retired covert operations officer with the Central Intelligence Agency (CIA). His career lead him to far-flung places, adventure, friendship, and even a wife he "recruited" in the Congo. As an intelligence officer in the world of espionage, he hunted for sources and was hunted by others in turn. Since retirement he has mostly avoided hunting of any kind but kept busy building a barn, raising children and chickens, working as a job coach for the disabled, and teaching classes as a substitute teacher—the latter pursuit being probably his most challenging endeavor! The Foley family resides in Utah.